ABC OF
SEXUALLY TRANSMITTED DISEASES

Fourth edition

ABC OF
SEXUALLY
TRANSMITTED DISEASES

FOURTH EDITION

MICHAEL W ADLER

Professor of Genitourinary Medicine,
University College London Medical School

with contributions from

IAN WELLER, RICHARD GILSON, IAN WILLIAMS, DAVID GOLDMEIER

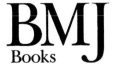

First published in 1984
by the BMJ Publishing Group, BMA House, Tavistock Square,
London WC1H 9JR

British Library Cataloguing in Publication Data

A catalogue record for this book is available from the
British Library

ISBN 0-7279-1368-9

First Edition 1984
Second Edition 1990
Third Edition 1995
Fourth Edition 1999

Typeset by Apek Typesetters, Nailsea, Bristol
Printed in Singapore by Craft Print Pte Ltd.

Contents

Acknowledgments

I am grateful to a number of my colleagues who have commented on various parts of the book as it was being written. I am particularly grateful to Drs RS Morton and T Moss, who read and commented on every one of the original articles prior to their appearance in the BMJ. I would also like to thank Dr JS Bingham, Dr D Harris, Dr F Cowan, the late Dr G Levine, Professor A Mindel, Dr JD Oriel, Professor Peckham, Dr G Ridgway, Dr J Sherrard and the late Dr RR Wilcox for their comments on individual chapters, and the Communicable Disease Surveillance Centre for allowing me to use some of their data. I would also like to thank colleagues who have allowed me to use their photographic material (Drs A Attenburrow, J Bingham and M Waugh), and the photographic department of University College London Medical School for their help. Finally, I thank my personal assistant, Alison Humphrey, who has shown great patience and skill throughout the whole of this project.

Michael W Adler

A CHANGING AND GROWING PROBLEM

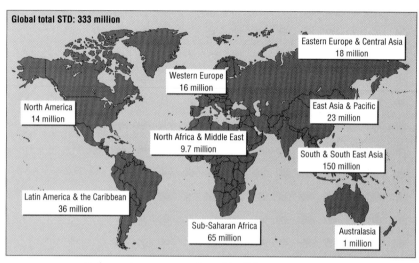

Estimated new cases of curable STD among adults

Estimated prevalence and incidence of STDs by region

Region	Prevalence per/1000	Incidence per/1000
Sub-Saharan Africa	208	254
South and South-East Asia	128	160
Latin America and Caribbean	95	145
Eastern Europe and Central Asia	75	112
North America	52	91
Australasia	52	91
Western Europe	45	77
Northern Africa and Middle East	40	60
East Asia and Pacific	19	28
Total	85	113

Sexually transmitted diseases (STDs) represent a major public health problem, and are among the commonest causes of illness, and even death, in the world and have far-reaching health, social and economic consequences. Failure to diagnose and treat traditional infections such as gonorrhoea, chlamydia and syphilis can have a deleterious effect on pregnancy and the newborn, eg miscarriage, prematurity, congenital and neonatal infections and blindness. Other complications, particularly in women, such as pelvic inflammatory disease, ectopic pregnancy, infertility and cervical cancer are large health and social problems. The World Health Organisation has estimated that there are approximately 333 million new cases of curable STDs per annum, of which 65 million occur in Sub-Saharan Africa and 150 million in South-East Asia. The incidence and prevalence of STD is highest in developing countries. The problem is costly to individuals and healthcare systems. It is estimated that for women aged 15–44 years the STDs, excluding HIV, are the second commonest cause of healthy life lost after maternal mobidity and mortality. The advent of HIV infection has highlighted the importance of infection spread by the sexual route.

In the United Kingdom the number of cases seen in sexually transmitted disease clinics (now known as departments of genitourinary medicine) has doubled over the past 20 years and now amounts to just over 900 000 new cases a year. For this reason sexually transmitted diseases need to be suspected and investigated in any patient who presents with what might at first look like a common clinical problem, such as a vaginal discharge, urinary tract infection, rash, or pelvic pain.

What are they?

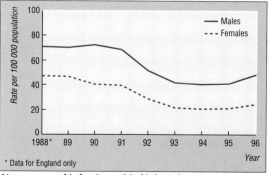

New cases of infection with *Neisseria gonorrhoeae* seen at GUM clinics: England and Wales 1988–96

The three commonest sexually transmitted diseases seen in clinics in 1996 (latest figures) are genital warts (97 240), non-gonococcal/non-specific urethritis (45 868), and chlamydial infection (31 857). Since the early 1970s there has been a steady decline in gonorrhoea, however in the last two years we have seen a slight increase in both sexes. For example, between 1995 and 1996 there was a 20% increase in both males (from 6471 to 7749 cases), and in females (from 3265 to 3902). Syphilis is not now a major problem and the small rise in the incidence of syphilis (mainly primary and secondary) in the 1970s and early 1980s has occurred mainly in homosexuals. The recent decline is probably accounted for by the adoption of safer sex techniques among this group with the advent of HIV infection and AIDS.

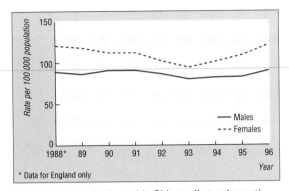

New cases of infection with *Chlamydia trachomatis* seen at GUM clinics: England and Wales 1988–96. Reproduced with permission from the PHLS Communicable Diseases Surveillance Centre *Communicable Diseases Report* 1997;7:44.

Trichomoniasis, pediculosis pubis, and genital herpes are common and are sexually transmitted. On the other hand, scabies and vaginal candidiasis are often diagnosed in sexually transmitted disease clinics, although they are not usually acquired sexually. Similarly, sexually transmitted hepatitis (A, B, and C) is becoming more common, and recently those working in clinics have become aware of the possible sexual transmission of β haemolytic streptococci, cytomegalovirus, and enteric pathogens. The Human Immunodeficiency virus (HIV) is the most recent condition to be spread sexually.

Among a wide variety of other conditions presenting to clinics, and requiring specialist investigation and treatment, are urinary tract infections, pelvic inflammatory disease, dermatological and psychosexual problems as well as patients with a morbid fear of sexually transmitted diseases. Chancroid, granuloma inguinale, lymphogranuloma venereum, yaws, and pinta are now rare in Britain. Finally, many patients seek reassurance, require simple counselling or advice, screening for HIV, and want general STD check ups; all need to be investigated. Approximately 117 000 people per year are tested for HIV in clinics.

Why have they increased?

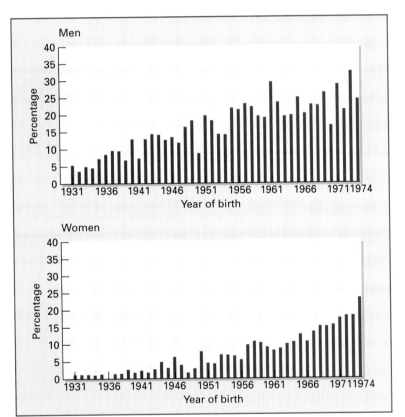

Proportion of men and women having first intercourse before 16 years of age by year of birth (From: *Sexual Attitudes and Lifestyle*. Blackwell)

Like many other medicosocial conditions—for example, suicide, alcoholism, cancer, and heart disease—the explanation for the increase in the sexually transmitted diseases is multifactorial.

The age of sexual maturity has decreased, the age at which people have sexual intercourse for the first time is lower, and more people have premarital sexual intercourse than previously. None of these indicate promiscuity, but it must be a factor. Also, the increasing use of the oral contraceptive pill and intrauterine devices has removed the protective effect of barrier techniques such as the sheath.

Because of the greatly improved service offered by the clinics and their ability to trace sexual contacts more people are seeking treatment who may not have previously done so. Thus how much of the increase in the number of recorded cases reflects a real or apparent trend is unknown.

Since populations are now more mobile nationally and internationally certain groups (tourists, professional travellers, members of the armed forces, immigrants) are at risk. They are separated from their families and social restraints and are more likely to have sexual contact outside a stable relationship.

Over the years the partial resistance of the gonococcus to penicillin has increased in many countries so that higher and higher curative doses have had to be used.

The final factor in the increasing incidence is the lack of resources for both good treatment facilities and coordinated research. Many countries still do not accept the importance of an open access, free service for sexually transmitted diseases, and even those countries with this facility often provide it in poor and old premises.

In developing countries, the role played by poverty, urbanisation, migration, social unrest, war, and the lack of diagnostic and treatment facilities, are more important than in the developed world.

How do they present?

Common presenting symptoms

Urethral discharge
Genital ulceration
Vaginal discharge +/− vulval irritation

The three commonest presenting symptoms are urethral discharge, genital ulceration, and vaginal discharge with or without vulval irritation. The descriptions in later chapters of the many diseases that may be spread sexually will show that patients may present with other symptoms (rash, dysuria, jaundice, arthralgia, rectal discharge). Additionally, several diseases may present initially with complications (abdominal or scrotal pain, urinary retention). Since they may affect any system in the body they should not be regarded solely as diseases of the genitals. Finally, the diseases are not always acute; many chronic conditions of the genital tract require long term management—for example, pelvic pain, recurrent herpes genitalis, and vaginal candidiasis.

How should they be managed?

Management

- Sexual history
- Physical examination
- Microbiology
- Serology
- Tracing sexual contacts
- Education
- Reassurance
- Follow up

The most important aspects of management are accurate diagnosis and effective treatment. Diagnosis needs time and skill in taking a detailed sexual history from both the patient and his or her sexual contacts and in carrying out a comprehensive physical examination. But above all microbiological and serological facilities are essential initially and at follow up for all patients to differentiate between the various diseases, exclude more than one occurring at a time, and identify asymptomatic disease. Some doctors have the facilities to perform some microbiological tests in their surgeries, but if not, referral to a clinic is strongly advised. These clinics now have a much more relaxed image and offer the patient a chance to seek help and advice with complete confidence and confidentiality. Strategies for management in resource-poor countries where specialist services are not available are covered in Chapter 18.

To prevent the spread of sexually transmitted diseases treatment must be effective and be seen to be effective. This means selecting the correct drug for the disease, carefully monitoring its administration, and carrying out regular follow up microbiological tests. The patient's sexual contacts must be traced so that they can be treated and thus prevent the disease from spreading further. The doctor may also play an important part in controlling the diseases by advising patients how best to avoid them, to recognise them, and to have them treated and by offering the opportunity for routine check ups for those who have put themselves at risk or who simply want reassurance. All of these facilities are offered within departments of genitourinary medicine.

Micro-organisms that can be sexually transmitted

Bacteria:
  Chlamydia trachomatis
  Neisseria gonorrhoeae
  Gardnerella vaginalis
  Treponema pallidum
  Group B haemolytic
    streptococcus
  Haemophilus ducreyi
  Calymmatobacterium
    granulomatis
  Shigella species
Mycoplasmas:
  Ureaplasma urealyticum
  Mycoplasma hominis
Parasites:
  Sarcoptes scabiei
  Phthirus pubis

Viruses:
  Herpes simplex virus
    types 1 and 2
  Wart virus
    (papillomavirus)
  Molluscum contagiosum
    virus (poxvirus)
  Hepatitis A, B and C virus
  Cytomegalovirus
  Human immunodeficiency
    virus 1 and 2
Protozoa:
  Entamoeba histolytica
  Giardia lamblia
  Trichomonas vaginalis
Fungi:
  Candida albicians

The workload of specialists in genitourinary medicine is continually increasing. Firstly, this is due to the realisation over the years that more and more diseases may be spread sexually, a point vividly illustrated recently by the epidemic of HIV infection and AIDS. Secondly, it is appreciated that other acute and chronic non-sexually acquired conditions are being managed in clinics. Genitourinary medicine is now a specialty in its own right, offering total care of people with a wide variety of conditions. The increased breadth of the speciality, and the knowledge that many patients seen in clinics do not have a sexually transmitted disease, have helped to reduce the stigma attached to clinics and should be of help to general practitioners, gynaecologists, and others wishing to refer patients for specialist advice.

URETHRAL DISCHARGE: DIAGNOSIS

The commonest presenting symptom of a sexually transmitted disease in men

A urethral discharge is the commonest presenting symptom of a sexually transmitted disease in men. A few discharges may be physiological but most are pathological; most of those seen by both general practitioners and specialists are pathological.

Causes

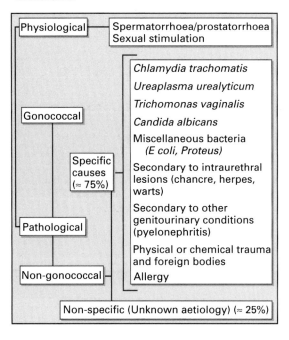

Broadly, pathological discharges are either gonococcal, due to infection with *Neisseria gonorrhoeae*, or non-gonococcal. The commonest cause of non-gonococcal urethritis is *Chlamydia trachomatis*, but it may also be due to infection with *Ureaplasma urealyticum*, *Trichomonas vaginalis*, or *Candida albicans* and sometimes to intraurethral lesions such as herpes genitalis, warts, or a syphilitic chancre. All these infections are acquired sexually. Rarely, pyelonephritis or a urinary tract infection may produce a urethral discharge. Attempts at intraurethral self medication with chemicals may cause a discharge, as may trauma from the use of sexual aids or the self inflicted lesions of dermatitis artefacta.

In about a quarter of cases of non-gonococcal urethritis no cause or infective agent may be identified, and these may be designated as true non-specific urethritis. Usually these discharges are assumed to be caused by a sexually transmitted infection which requires treatment.

Small amounts of clear or mucoid urethral discharge after sexual intercourse are probably the result of sexual stimulation. In the absence of sexual arousal the discharge may be due to spermatorrhoea or prostatorrhoea, both of which may be noticed at urination or defecation.

Taking a history

History/important features of urethral discharge

- Site: urethral/subpreputial
- Colour: yellow or white, clear or profuse
- Duration
- Note: 5–10% of patients with gonococcal or non-gonococcal urethritis have no symptoms

An accurate history must be taken, particularly of the clinical features and sexual factors, and a physical examination and full microbiological tests performed.

Clinical features—When a patient complains of a discharge it is important to identify its site. Uncircumcised men may develop a subpreputial infection (for example, herpetic or candidal) or disease (for example, inflammation from smegma or trauma, skin disorders, or malignancy) but find it difficult to pinpoint the exact source of the discharge. The patient may describe the colour and quantity of the discharge as yellow, white, clear, profuse, scanty, or a combination of these. Such descriptions give little indication of the type of infective agent present. Likewise, the fact that the incubation period of gonorrhoea (two to five days) is often shorter than for chlamydial or other types of non-gonococcal infection (seven to 14 days) should not be used to make a non-microbiological clinical diagnosis. Five to 10% of patients with gonococcal or non-gonococcal urethritis have no symptoms.

Sexual factors—Details of the number and type of sexual contacts in the previous four weeks and whether or not the partner has symptoms or has been treated recently must be determined. If the patient is homosexual it is necessary to know which anatomical sites have been exposed to risk—for example, the rectum or the throat as well as the urethra or a combination of all three. More than one site may be affected, and appropriate tests on samples from the rectum, throat or both—as well as from the urethra—may be needed. Because of the development of strains of *N gonorrhoeae* that are resistant to penicillin, details of sexual contact in other countries must be obtained. In all cases contact tracing of sexual contacts needs to be carried out to determine the source of the infection and the people who may in turn have been infected by the patient.

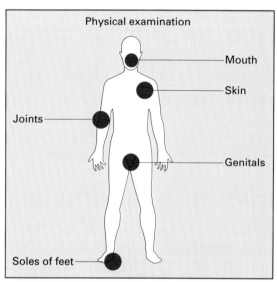

Sexual history

- Homosexual or heterosexual
- Number of partners
- Symptoms in partner(s)
- Overseas contact
- Sites of contact

Physical examination

Physical examination

- Mouth
- Skin
- Joints
- Genitals
- Soles of feet

The penis should be thoroughly examined, particularly with the prepuce retracted, as should the scrotum and its contents, the pubic hair and surrounding skin, and the perianal area. The physical examination should not be limited to the genitals since with a "fly button" approach important information may be missed. A thorough general physical examination is needed to exclude possible complications of gonorrhoea or non-gonococcal infection. Often patients have more than one sexually transmitted disease at a time, and these may be missed unless the patient is comprehensively examined. Particular attention should be paid to the skin, soles of the feet, mouth, and joints. The need to undertake a detailed physical examination is illustrated by HIV infection and AIDS, which can present in virtually any system of the body.

A specimen of urethral discharge must be collected for Gram staining and microscopical examination. The slides may be stained immediately and a presumptive diagnosis of gonococcal or non-gonococcal urethritis made. Gonorrhoea will be confirmed by the presence of Gram negative intracellular diplococci, whereas non-gonococcal urethritis will be confirmed by their absence but the presence of ≥5 polymorphonuclear leucocytes per high power field (×1000 magnification). *C trachomatis* cannot, however, be identified by direct microscopy.

T vaginalis is not a common cause of urethral discharge and is probably worth looking for only in patients with chronic urethritis and those whose female sexual contacts already have trichomoniasis. A specimen of discharge is placed on a slide (with one drop of saline), a coverslip added, and examined without staining under the microscope with dark ground illumination.

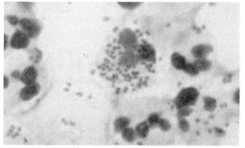

Culture

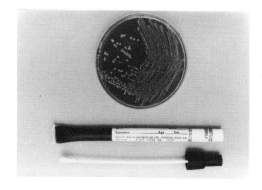

As up to 10% of cases of gonorrhoea may be missed if microscopy alone forms the basis of diagnosis, specimens of urethral discharge should ideally be cultured for *N gonorrhoeae*. The discharge may be plated directly on to a selective medium—for example, Thayer-Martin or modified New York City medium—which has added antibiotics to suppress overgrowth by other micro-organisms. The plates are incubated at 36°C in an enriched carbon dioxide environment (5–10%) for 48 hours in candle extinction jars or a carbon dioxide incubator. If a transport medium is needed, either Stuart's or Amies's may be used, but specimens must reach the laboratory for plating out (as above) within 24 hours. Confirmatory tests, such as oxidase reaction, sugar fermentation, or coagglutination on suspected cultures help to distinguish *N gonorrhoeae* from other organisms.

Although the most specific test for *C. trachomatis* is cell culture, facilities are no longer widely available in the United Kingdom.

Antigen detection tests, such as direct immunofluorescence and enzyme immunoassay which use polyclonal or monoclonal antibodies, are readily available. The sensitivity of enzyme immunoassays has been questioned with the advent of sensitive nucleic acid detection based tests. Polymerase or ligase chain reaction (PCR/LCR) testing is now established as the optimal methodology. Other techniques, such as transcription mediated amplification (TMA) are also available, but require further evaluation. These tests have the advantage that they can be used on urine specimens from either sex, and also low vaginal swabs, suggesting that in the future an invasive test may be unnecessary. For medicolegal purposes, culture of the organism is to be preferred.

Blood and urine tests

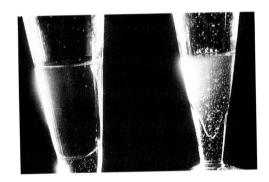

A urine sample should be collected. In the two glass urine test the patient is asked to pass about 60–120 ml into the first glass (first voided urine) and the remainder of his specimen into the second. The presence of threads or specks of pus and a hazy appearance which is not due to phosphates—that is, it does not clear after 5–10% acetic acid has been added—in the first glass confirms anterior urethritis. This test may easily be carried out by the general practitioner before referral and will help to differentiate an anterior from a posterior urethritis, a cystitis, or a nephritis (hazy urine with threads in both glasses). The referring practitioner should advise the patient to hold his urine for at least four hours before attending the clinic; this allows for the discharge to collect within the urethra. Some patients who give a history of discharge have no evidence of this when examined. In these cases it may be worth while repeating the investigations after the patient has held his urine overnight.

Blood samples should be collected from all patients to exclude concurrent infection with syphilis and an anti-HIV antibody test offered and discussed.

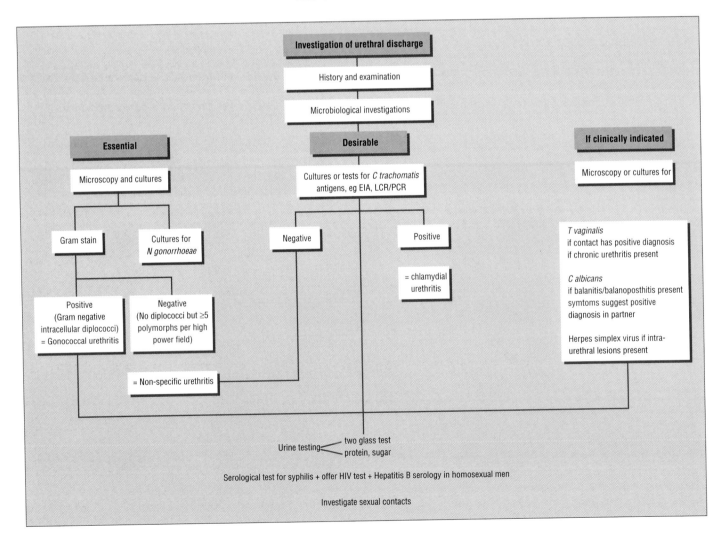

URETHRAL DISCHARGE: MANAGEMENT

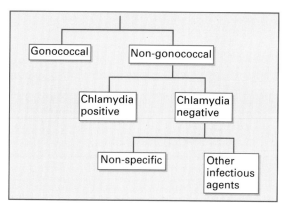

Gonococcal urethritis

Chemotherapy

Ampicillin
Amoxycillin

If allergic to penicillin:
  Ciprofloxacin
  Spectinomycin
  Tetracycline

Since the treatment of a gonococcal urethritis differs fundamentally from that for non-gonococcal urethritis an accurate microbiological diagnosis is essential, as are repeated microbiological tests at follow up. For this reason, and because of the need to exclude concurrent infections and trace sexual contacts, many doctors may prefer their patients to attend their local department of genitourinary medicine after initial physical examination and investigation and investigations in the surgery (see box).

Penicillin is the drug of choice and whereas in the past was usually given intramuscularly is now mostly given as an oral preparation. The most commonly used within the United Kingdom is ampicillin/amoxycyllin 3 g in a single dose plus 1 g of probenecid. Patients with genital gonorrhoea are often given a course of tetracycline in case of concomitant chlamydial infection. This should start the day after initial treatment with penicillin. The usual regimen that can be used is doxycycline 100 mg twice a day for one week. If tetracyclines are contraindicated, erythromycin stearate 500 mg twice a day for 14 days can be used.

If the patient is allergic to penicillin then ciprofloxacin 500 mg by mouth may be given, spectinomycin 2 g intramuscularly, doxycycline 100 mg twice a day for 7 days, or tetracycline 500 mg by mouth every six hours for 7 days. Ciprofloxacin should not be used in pregnant patients or those with a history of convulsions. In these situations spectinomycin is the preferable alternative. Because ciprofloxacin is not treponemicidal it may be given to those patients being

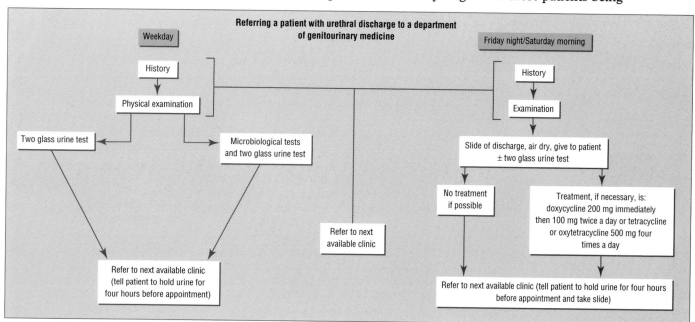

investigated for suspected syphilis. These regimens are suggested for use only in the United Kingdom. Regimens in other countries will depend on the sensitivities of the gonococcus, the availability of antibiotics, and the ability to follow up the patient after treatment. Since patients may not return some countries advocate the use of tetracycline in the treatment of gonorrhoea since it will eradicate *N gonorrhoeae* as well as concurrent infection with *Chlamydia trachomatis*.

Follow-up—Within three to seven days after treatment the patient should have further microbiological tests of cure (smears and cultures) carried out. He should be advised to abstain from further sexual contact until this follow up visit. All sexual contacts should be encouraged to attend a clinic or their general practitioner for investigation and treatment. Ideally, serological tests for syphilis should be carried out for all patients after three months, as the initial investigations may have become positive by the end of the full incubation period of this condition. Tests for HIV should also be offered.

> **Advice and follow up**
>
> Avoid sexual intercourse
> Investigate and treat sexual contacts
> Repeat smears and cultures 7 days
>   after treatment
> Test blood samples for syphilis ± HIV at
>   3 months

Treatment failure

> **Treatment failure**
>
> Reinfection:
>   Penicillin
> Resistant infections:
>   Spectinomycin
>   Ciprofloxacin
> Postgonococcal urethritis:
>   Doxycycline/tetracycline

If patients with a gonococcal urethritis do not respond to penicillin and still harbour *N gonorrhoeae* two possibilities need to be considered: reinfection or infection with a penicillinase producing strain of *N gonorrhoeae*. Reinfection needs further treatment with penicillin whereas an infection due to a resistant strain of *N gonorrhoeae* must be treated with spectinomycin 2 g intramuscularly or ciprofloxacin 500 mg orally.

Some patients (25–50%) in whom a concurrent course of tetracycline has not been used develop a postgonococcal urethritis after treatment with penicillin. This is caused by *C trachomatis* in 80% of cases. Doxycycline 100 mg twice a day for seven days should be given or tetracycline 500 mg should be given every six hours for seven days. If the discharge persists the same regimen should be continued for a further seven days.

Non-gonococcal urethritis

> **Chemotherapy**
>
> ● Doxycycline
> ● Tetracycline
> ● Oxytetracycline
> ● Erythromycin stearate

Chemotherapy—Fortunately, the same treatment regimen is effective in both chlamydia positive and chlamydia negative non-gonococcal urethritis. The tetracyclines are the antibiotic of first choice, usually doxycycline 100 mg twice a day for seven days or tetracycline/ oxytetracycline 500 mg six hourly for seven days. A second-choice treatment for patients allergic to tetracycline, or pregnant, is erythromycin stearate 500 mg twice a day for 14 days. Newer drugs, such as azithromycin, can be used, it has the advantage of being given as a stat dose, but is expensive. The patient should be advised to avoid sexual intercourse and milk products.

Follow up—Even though a one week course of a tetracycline is effective in curing both chlamydia positive and chlamydia negative non-gonococcal urethritis, patient compliance and drug absorption have to be perfect for this to occur. Thus after one week of treatment the patient should be seen so that compliance, side effects, and clinical progress can be assessed. If the urethritis has not responded after one week of treatment erythromycin stearate 500 mg should be given 12 hourly for 14 days plus metronidazole 2 grams stat. The sexual contacts of all patients undergoing treatment must be investigated and treated. Unfortunately, this is sometimes overlooked until it becomes clear that the patient with persistent infection is being reinfected by his partner(s). Finally, a patient with non-gonococcal urethritis should ideally be investigated for syphilis after three months and HIV if necessary.

On occasions the urethritis becomes chronic and further investigations—for example, of the prostate—will be needed. All too often, however, these patients are not suffering from infective urethritis but have become anxious self examiners and "squeezers," a condition reinforced by inexperienced doctors who treat the microscope slide and not the whole patient.

Other infective agents only rarely give rise to a urethral discharge; those due to *T vaginalis*, *C albicans*, warts, herpes simplex virus, syphilitic chancre, and trauma are covered in later chapters.

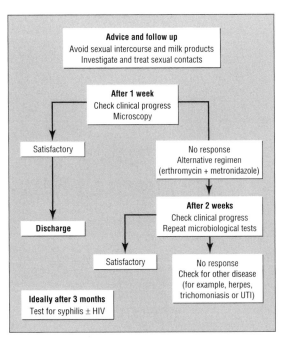

VAGINAL DISCHARGE: DIAGNOSIS

Vaginal discharge is a common presenting symptom seen by general practitioners, gynaecologists, and those working in family planning clinics and departments of genitourinary medicine. As with urethral discharge, vaginal discharge may be either physiological or pathological in origin. It is difficult to know what proportion of discharges belong to either category since there have been few community based prevalence studies.

Physiological causes—Vaginal discharge is a continuum, and as such the concept of normality does not exist. Some patients have a copious discharge, others none or little. Only the patient can, therefore, determine what is her own normal experience. It is worthwhile reminding patients that a normal vaginal discharge may increase and be noticed only premenstrually, at the time of ovulation, or when using the contraceptive pill or an intrauterine device. Non-pathological lesions on the cervix such as ectropion can cause a discharge.

Pathological (infective) causes—The commonest organism giving rise to an infective pathological vaginal discharge is *Candida albicans*. Other causes of this symptom include vaginal infections with *Trichomonas vaginalis*, bacterial vaginosis, and anaerobic organisms, and cervical infections with *Neisseria gonorrhoeae* and *Chlamydia trachomatis*. Cervical lesions due to herpes, warts, and a syphilitic chancre may also cause a discharge. There is some doubt about whether *Ureaplasma urealyticum* and haemolytic streptococci do cause a vaginal discharge, and the discharge of the rare toxic shock syndrome is usually coincidental and overshadowed by the patient's general condition.

Pathological (non-infective) causes—Localised cervical lesions such as polyps and neoplasms may present with a vaginal discharge. It is surprising what may be retained in the vagina without the patient's knowledge: tampons and the occasional condom are common, but cloves of garlic have also been found. Trauma may be caused by sexual aids and irritant substances.

Pathological causes

Infective:
  Candida albicans
  Trichomonas vaginalis
  Bacterial vaginosis
  Anaerobic organisms
  Chlamydia trachomatis
  Neisseria gonorrhoeae
  Cervical herpes genitalis
  Cervical warts
  Syphilitic chancre
  Toxic shock syndrome
    (*? Staphylococcus aureus*)
  Mycoplasmas
  β haemolytic streptococci

Non-infective:
  Cervical ectropion
  Cervical polyp(s)
  Neoplasm
  Retained products
    (tampon, postabortion, postnatal)
  Trauma
  Allergy

History

As with urethral discharge, a careful history, physical examination, and microbiological tests are essential to establish an accurate diagnosis and to exclude a sexually acquired infection.

Certain points in the clinical history suggest that a sexually transmitted disease is a possibility—such as the development of symptoms after a recent change of sexual partner or recent multiple sexual contacts. Further points that should make the doctor suspect a sexually transmitted disease are symptoms in the patient that are recurrent or persistent and symptoms in her sexual partner. A urethral discharge in a woman's partner makes it highly likely that her symptoms are due to a sexually transmitted infection. Irritation, soreness, and redness of her partner's penis after sexual contact suggests infection with *Candida albicans*. Finally, the patient should be asked about any other symptoms that suggest complications of a sexually transmitted disease—for example, abdominal pain, rash, arthralgia, dyspareunia, or altered menstruation.

High risk profile

- Partner change
- Multiple contacts
- Recurrent symptoms
- Symptoms in partner
- General symptoms:
    Abdominal pain
    Menstrual problems
    Rash
    Dyspareunia
    Arthralgia

Neither the patient's symptoms nor a subjective description of the colour and quality of the discharge are of much value in reaching an accurate diagnosis. Even more so than in men genitourinary symptoms in women are a poor guide to the exact nature of the condition.

Physical and laboratory investigations

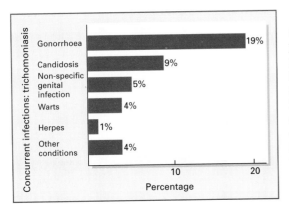

If a sexually transmitted disease is suspected from the clinical and sexual history the patient should be examined fully to exclude possible complications and coincidental abnormalities. Once the physical examination has been carried out local genital examination and tests should be undertaken. As with the symptoms, the physical signs and macroscopic appearance of a vaginal discharge do not help in making an accurate diagnosis. For instance, to rely on the suggestion that the discharge of vaginal candidiasis is thick, curdy, and white will result in the wrong diagnosis in most instances. Similarly, no reliance should be placed on the supposed association between a frothy greenish discharge and trichomoniasis.

Infection can be diagnosed accurately only after microbiological tests have been carried out on samples from the appropriate anatomical sites. Women attending departments of genitourinary medicine have tests performed routinely to establish or exclude a diagnosis of candidiasis, trichomoniasis, bacterial vaginosis, gonorrhoea, and *Chlamydia trachomatis* infection. So that samples may be obtained from the appropriate sites a speculum should be passed to visualise accurately the cervix, posterior fornix, and the vagina. The reason these tests are performed routinely is because sexually transmitted diseases may occur concurrently. In clinics one fifth of the cases of trichomoniasis are associated with gonorrhoea.

Candida albicans may be excluded by microscopy of a Gram stained smear and by culture of material from the vaginal wall. Both cells and mycelia stain Gram positive. Since some cases may be missed when microscopy alone is relied on, cultures should be carried out to confirm the diagnosis or they may be used alone without microscopy. Traditionally, cultures are plated on Sabouraud's medium and incubated at 37°C for 48 hours; Stuart's or Amies's transport medium may be used when necessary. Other yeasts—for example, *Torulopsis glabrata*—also occasionally inhabit the female genital tract and grow on culture. Definitive differentiation may be achieved only by additional tests. *Trichomonas vaginalis* is usually best isolated from the posterior fornix, and a wet preparation using a drop of saline should be examined immediately by dark ground microscopy. Though the diagnosis may be confirmed by culture, microscopy alone is extremely reliable. The specimen of discharge must be placed directly into Feinberg-Whittington medium and incubated for 48 hours at 37°C or sent to the laboratories in Stuart's or Amies's transport media. Feinberg–Whittington can also be used to culture *Candida albicans*.

Gonorrhoea is an infection of mucous membranes, and since the vagina is lined with stratified squamous epithelium a high vaginal swab is not the best method of sampling in diagnosing this condition. The most productive sites for isolating the gonococcus are the endocervix and the urethra. Specimens should be taken from both sites, Gram stained, and cultured. As with specimens of urethral discharge the culture material may be put into a suitable transport medium (for example, Stuart's) or plated directly and incubated. Gram stained microcopy for *Neisseria gonorrhoeae* in women is unreliable. Reliance on this alone results in about a half of cases being missed. All women in whom gonorrhoea is suspected should therefore have cultures performed in addition to microscopy. One set of smears and cultures should detect 90% of cases. This figure may be increased by repeat testing and by sampling other sites.

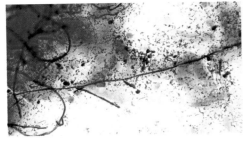

Mycelia

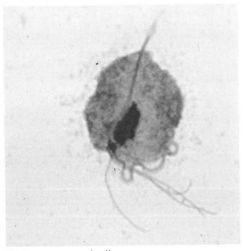

Trichomonas vaginalis

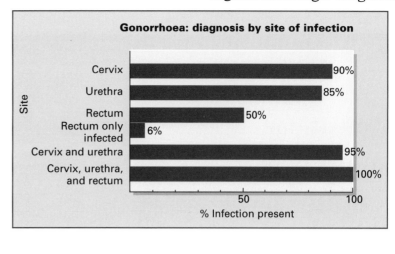

Gonorrhoea

- Samples from:
  Urethra
  Endocervix
  Rectum (for sexual
  contacts of men
  with gonorrhoea)
  Pharynx (if oral intercourse)
- Microscopy (Gram
  stained smear)
- Culture

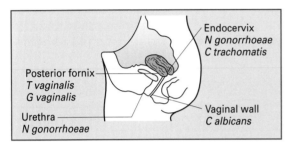

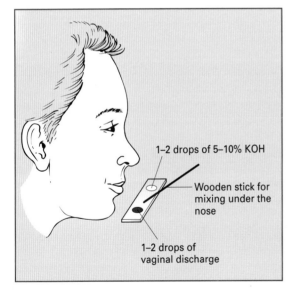

The gonococcus may be isolated from the rectum in women with gonorrhoea in about 6% of cases in which it is not found in the conventional sites, the cervix and urethra. Proctitis arises more often by autoinoculation from vaginal discharge than from anal intercourse. For this reason all women who are contacts of men with gonorrhoea should have rectal tests carried out in the hope of increasing the chances of isolating the gonococcus. In addition, pharyngeal cultures for *N gonorrhoeae* should be taken in those women who report oral intercourse.

C trachomatis is an important sexually transmitted agent which often causes asymptomatic infections and may occur concurrently with other sexually acquired agents, in particular *N gonorrhoeae*. An endocervical specimen should be taken for *C trachomatis* in any woman attending a clinic.

Vaginal discharge can also occur as a result of bacterial vaginosis. Certain clinical and diagnostic features seem to be associated with this infection: a fishy smelling discharge, which is particularly noticeable after sexual intercourse; the presence of clue cells (bacteria attached to vaginal epithelial cells) in a drop of infected discharge mixed with saline and viewed under the microscope; a pH of the vaginal discharge $\geqslant 4.5$ (easily measured by pH paper); and a positive result on the amine test. This test is performed by adding one to two drops of discharge and 5–10% potassium hydroxide together on a glass slide. If a fishy ammoniacal odour is released the result is positive. A similar smell may be obtained when *T vaginalis* or spermatozoa are present in the vaginal discharge. Bacterial vaginosis and a mixture of anaerobes—for example, *Bacteroides* spp, peptococci, peptostreptococci, mobiluncus—are usually found in high concentrations in patients with bacterial vaginosis. Diagnosis is made on the above criteria without the need for culture.

Finally, all patients should have serological tests for syphilis carried out to exclude this as a concurrent infection and be offered an HIV test. Urine should be tested for protein and glucose, and cervical cytology if not performed in the previous three years.

Isolation rate for *C trachomatis*

Gonorrhoea contacts	30–60%
Non-gonococcal urethritis contacts	30–35%
Attending GUM clinics (excluding above groups)	2–17%
Attending family planning/well woman clinics	2–7%

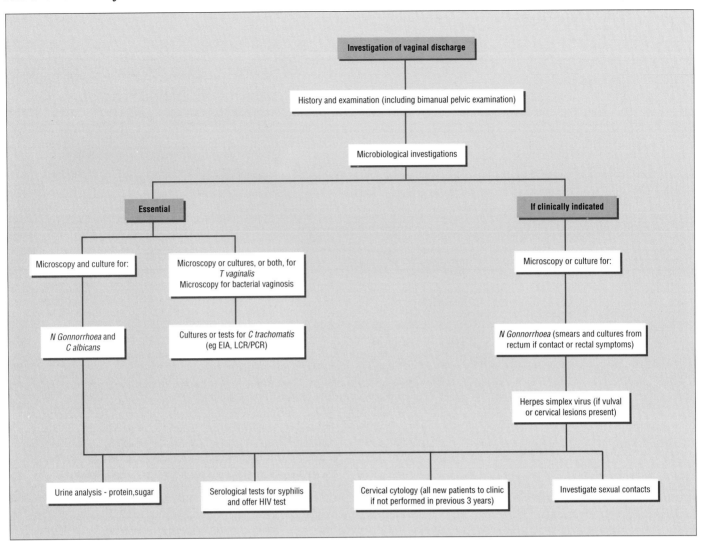

Investigation of vaginal discharge

History and examination (including bimanual pelvic examination)

Microbiological investigations

Essential

If clinically indicated

Microscopy and culture for:

Microscopy or cultures, or both, for
T vaginalis
Microscopy for bacterial vaginosis

Microscopy or culture for:

N Gonnorrhoea and
C albicans

Cultures or tests for *C trachomatis*
(eg EIA, LCR/PCR)

N Gonnorrhoea (smears and cultures from
rectum if contact or rectal symptoms)

Herpes simplex virus (if vulval
or cervical lesions present)

Urine analysis - protein,sugar

Serological tests for syphilis
and offer HIV test

Cervical cytology (all new patients to clinic
if not performed in previous 3 years)

Investigate sexual contacts

VAGINAL DISCHARGE: MANAGEMENT

Vaginal candidiasis

Despite the introduction of new oral antifungal agents (ketoconazole, itraconazole, and fluconazole), the cornerstone of the treatment of vaginal candidiasis is still intravaginal pessaries. Imidazole preparations (clotrimazole, miconazole, econazole) need only be prescribed for short periods—for example, clotrimazole pessaries 500 mg once at night or 200 mg nightly for three days. Vulval irritation may be relieved by local nystatin or clotrimazole cream applied twice a day.

The condition may recur, and it is always worth explaining simple methods of genital hygiene and the possible precipitating factors to the patient at the time of her initial attack, since this may help the condition to resolve and prevent recurrences. The patient should be advised to keep the genital area clean, dry, and untraumatised, ideally by not wearing nylon pants, tights, or jeans. Since autoinfection from the bowel may occur, cleaning with toilet paper should be in a backwards direction.

Predisposing factors—Trauma to the vaginal mucosa may predispose to infection and may occur during intercourse or when vaginal deodorants, perfumed soaps, and bubble baths are used. The patient may require additional lubrication with K-Y jelly during sexual intercourse. Pregnancy, antibiotics, corticosteroid and immunosuppressive treatment, diabetes, orogenital contact, and the presence of other sexually transmitted diseases have all been implicated in both initial and recurrent disease. The sexual partner may occasionally be the source of infection and reinfection.

Follow-up—If possible patients should be seen at least once after treatment to assess the clinical and microbiological response and so that any other treatment may be started if additional sexually acquired infections have been identified in the laboratory after the initial set of tests at first consultation.

Treatment of relapsing infection—A relapse shortly after initial treatment needs a longer course of treatment—for example, if clotrimazole is used 100 mg should be given daily for 12 days. If this regimen fails an increased dose of 200 mg daily should be given for 12 days. Prophylactic treatment may be tried with clotrimazole 500 mg once a week or monthly for two to three months. A small number of women will have recurrent candidiasis (four or more episodes per year), and in these patients, predisposing risk factors should be excluded. Oral antifungals can be used as a maintenance suppressive regimen. For example, six months of ketoconazole 100 mg orally once daily, itraconazole 100–500 mg per day, and fluconazole 100 mg a week.

Sexual contacts—Candidiasis is not usually sexually transmitted but male contacts should be seen, firstly, if they have symptoms and, secondly, if the woman is having repeated recurrences. The man should be thoroughly investigated, as was his female partner, to make sure that he has no concurrent sexually transmitted disease, since this is likely to predispose to candidal infection. Candidal balanitis is treated with saline bathing and application of nystatin or clotrimazole cream.

Management

- Vaginal pessaries:
  Clotrimazole
  Miconazole
  Econazole
  Nystatin

- Genital hygiene:
  Clean
  Dry
  Avoid trauma or irritation

- Assess clinical and microbiological response

- Treat other infections/conditions

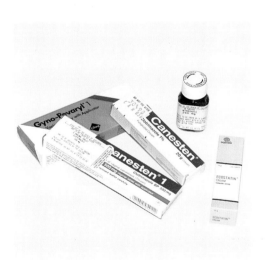

Trichomoniasis

Infection with *Trichomonas vaginalis* should be treated with a single dose of metronidazole 2 g. The patient should be warned of the possible disulfiram like (Antabuse) effect of these drugs in association with alcohol. Unless patients are warned they quite logically give up the tablets rather than the alcohol. Patients should be followed up at least once for microbiological tests of cure after treatment, and so that any other infections detected may be treated. Patients not responding to treatment should be given metronidazole 400 mg every 12 hours for seven days. Continued failure usually indicates that *(a)* the patient is being reinfected by her sexual partner; *(b)* she is not complying with the medication; *(c)* the drug is not being absorbed; or *(d)* it is being inhibited locally by vaginal bacteria. Sometimes patients need to be admitted to hospital for supervision of treatment. With recurrent/relapsing infection, other therapies can be considered such as betadine pessaries 250 mg twice a day intravaginally for two weeks, acetarsol pessaries 250 mg twice a day intravaginally for two weeks, or metronidazole suppositories inserted intravaginally 1 g twice a day for one week. Anecdotal reports have suggested that tinidazole can be useful at 2 g per day orally for 10 days. Its efficacy is not fully evaluated.

Management

- Clinical history

- Confirm by microbiological diagnosis

- Treat with metronidazole, avoid alcohol

- Follow up:
  Assess microbiological response
  Repeat treatment if necessary

- Investigate and treat sexual contacts

Treatment failure

- Reinfection

- Non-compliance

- Poor absorption

- Inhibition by vaginal bacteria

Treatment in pregnancy—Laboratory studies on animals have suggested that massive doses of metronidazole are teratogenic, even though this effect has not been reported in humans. It is therefore probably unwise to use it in the first trimester of pregnancy. Metronidazole may pass into breast milk and should therefore not be used during lactation.

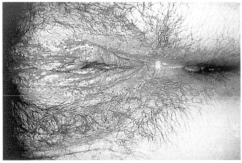
Candidal vulvovaginitis.

Since *T vaginalis* infestation is usually sexually acquired and often occurs concurrently with other sexually transmitted infections—for example, with gonorrhoea in approximately 20% of cases—it should never be treated without full microbiological investigations and examination of regular sexual contacts. The organism is extremely difficult to identify in the male urethra, and usually the contacts are given a course of metronidazole even if trichomonads cannot be detected after examination and testing (epidemiological treatment). This does not, however, imply that contacts should be treated by proxy. In view of the high incidence of associated infections all regular contacts should be seen and have microbiological tests performed.

Other infections

Both uncomplicated gonococcal and chlamydial infections in women are treated as for men (see previous chapter) with the same doses of penicillin or tetracycline. Female contacts of men with chlamydia negative non-gonococcal urethritis should be treated with tetracycline despite the absence of an organism. If the patient is using oral contraception and is being treated with a tetracycline, she should be warned to use extra precautions while on the drug, and for 7 days after finishing treatment. If the patient is pregnant, erythromycin stearate 500 mg twice a day for 14 days should be used instead of a tetracycline.

Bacterial vaginosis should be treated with metronidazole 2 g as a single dose, or metronidazole 400 mg twice daily for 5 days. Recurrent attacks in the female can be treated with further metronidazole, preferably a 5-day course. Clindamycin cream 2% intravaginally for 7 days can also be used. During the first trimester of pregnancy, metronidazole is contraindicated.

Because bacterial vaginosis has been associated with adverse outcomes of pregnancy, for example premature rupture of the membranes, preterm labour and birth, it is important that this infection is treated in the pregnant woman.

Routine treatment of sexual partners is not recommended because there is no scientific evidence that the likelihood of relapse or recurrence in the female is affected by the treatment of her sexual partner(s).

Management

- Uncomplicated gonorrhoea
  Penicillin

- Chlamydial infections
  Tetracycline

- Contacts of men with chlamydia negative non-gonococcal urethritis
  Tetracycline

- Anaerobic vaginosis
  Metronidazole

Management by the non-specialist

Epidemiological studies and ad hoc surveys of women attending gynaecology, obstetric, and family planning clinics indicate that candidiasis is more common than trichomoniasis, chlamydia, or gonorrhoea. Nevertheless, studies in departments of genitourinary medicine indicate that all these infections may occur concurrently. For these reasons non-specialists may adopt various methods of management of genitourinary symptoms, depending on their own circumstances and the availability of laboratory facilities.

The academic approach—Because the common conditions causing vaginal discharge with or without vulval irritation may occur concurrently microbiological specimens should ideally be taken from all patients presenting with vaginal discharge. A speculum should be passed and endocervical and vaginal specimens obtained (see previous chapter). If the doctor has a microscope and Gram staining facilities candidiasis, trichomoniasis, and gonorrhoea can be excluded. Microscopy is fallible in all of these infections and specimens should be sent to the laboratory. Unless a microscopic diagnosis is made treatment should be withheld until the results have returned from the laboratory.

The realistic approach would be to perform the tests as above but to start treatment at the first consultation on the basis of the patient's history, absence or presence and type of symptoms in the sexual partner(s), examination, and the knowledge that common things occur commonly—namely candidiasis. This course should be followed only if the doctor insists on a follow up visit to assess the patient's progress and determine whether the correct treatment has been given in the light of the microbiological results.

For both the academic and realistic approaches contact tracing is an essential aspect of managing a sexually acquired infection. Both the source of infection and those who may in turn have been infected by the patient should lee traced. Non-specialists often forget that for each patient sitting in front of them there are at least two others infected in the community.

The pragmatic approach—Vaginal discharge with or without vulval irritation is a common presenting symptom and is most often due to an infection with *Candida albicans*. Therefore empirical treatment may be given without microbiological confirmation. This approach is contrary to that practised by the genitourinary physician, and, although the ideal would be to carry out microbiological investigations on all patients, limitation of resources and time may preclude this. This approach is reasonable so long as three failsafe mechanisms are observed. Firstly, an accurate clinical and sexual history must be taken to identify the high risk patient who needs tests or referral (see previous chapter). Secondly, treat for candidiasis alone so as not to mask other infections. The third mechanism is to insist that the patient returns for follow up after treatment. If symptoms are still present a concurrent sexually transmitted disease or wrong initial diagnosis may be a possibility, and the patient will need microbiological tests or referral to a department of genitourinary medicine.

The pragmatic approach is treatment before diagnosis and is acceptable only for low risk patients who will return for reassessment after treatment.

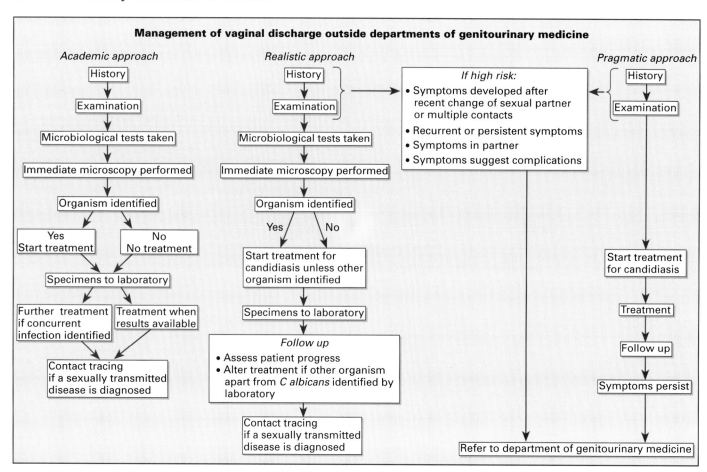

Management of vaginal discharge outside departments of genitourinary medicine

Academic approach

History → Examination → Microbiological tests taken → Immediate microscopy performed → Organism identified

Yes Start treatment / No No treatment → Specimens to laboratory

Further treatment if concurrent infection identified | Treatment when results available → Contact tracing if a sexually transmitted disease is diagnosed

Realistic approach

History → Examination → Microbiological tests taken → Immediate microscopy performed → Organism identified

Yes / No → Start treatment for candidiasis unless other organism identified → Specimens to laboratory → Follow up
• Assess patient progress
• Alter treatment if other organism apart from *C albicans* identified by laboratory
→ Contact tracing if a sexually transmitted disease is diagnosed

If high risk:
• Symptoms developed after recent change of sexual partner or multiple contacts
• Recurrent or persistent symptoms
• Symptoms in partner
• Symptoms suggest complications

Pragmatic approach

History → Examination → Start treatment for candidiasis → Treatment → Follow up → Symptoms persist

Refer to department of genitourinary medicine

COMPLICATIONS OF COMMON GENITAL INFECTIONS AND INFECTIONS IN OTHER SITES

	Infection		
		Chlamydia	
Complications	Gonococcal	Positive	Negative
Women			
Local: Pelvic inflammatory disease	+	+	+
Bartholinitis/abscess	+	–	–
Systemic: Disseminated infection	+	–	–
Men			
Local: Epididymitis/orchitis	+	+	+
Prostatitis (±vesiculitis)	+	+	+
Systemic: Reiter's disease	–	+	+
Disseminated infection	+	–	–

If patients are treated early complications rarely occur. When they arise they are usually associated with chlamydia positive or chlamydia negative non-gonococcal infections or gonorrhoea and may be local or systemic.

Local complications: pelvic inflammatory disease

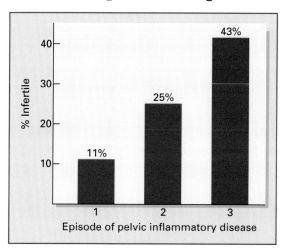

% Infertile vs Episode of pelvic inflammatory disease: 1 = 11%, 2 = 25%, 3 = 43%

Pelvic inflammatory disease (PID) is the most important complication associated with these three types of infection. About 10% of patients develop this complication after a gonococcal or non-gonococcal infection. In England and Wales the number of cases admitted to hospital has trebled in the past 25 years. In the United States the estimated direct costs of PID are $3200 m a year. In some African countries up to 50% of gynaecological admissions are due to this condition. In all of these countries many more cases are managed on an outpatient basis, for which no routine statistics are available.

Long term morbidity after recovery from acute PID is considerable: chronic abdominal pain, menstrual disturbances, dyspareunia, infertility, tubal pregnancy, medical consultation and medication, time off work, and psychological sequelae. The most disastrous consequence of salpingitis is sterility. The proportion of patients with salpingitis who develop tubal occlusion rises from 10% to 13% with a first attack to 75% with three or more.

The diagnosis of PID is often difficult. Clinically there is a combination of symptoms and signs, but even when these are correlated with laparoscopic findings the clinical diagnosis is correct in only 65% of patients. The condition is most often confused with appendicitis, endometriosis, and ectopic pregnancy.

Since acute PID is often the direct result of a sexually transmitted infection, full microbiological tests must be carried out to detect infection with *Chlamydia trachomatis* or *Neisseria gonorrhoeae*.

In all cases patients should be encouraged to rest in bed, even if they are not admitted to hospital. Any intrauterine device should be removed once treatment has started.

Pelvic inflammatory disease

Symptoms	Signs
Lower abdominal pain	Fever
Malaise	Abdominal tenderness
Vaginal discharge	Adnexal tenderness ±pelvic mass
Dyspareunia, dysmenorrhoea	Cervical motion tenderness
	Purulent cervical discharge

Indications for admission to hospital

- Diagnosis uncertain ? ectopic
                              pregnancy
                              ? appendicitis

- Severely ill

- Unable to rest at home (living alone,
                              young children)

- Unable to tolerate outpatient treatment

- Failure to respond to outpatient treatment

- Pregnant

Non-gonococcal salpingitis
tetracycline
        +
metronidazole

Gonococcal infections
ampicillin/amoxycillin (if penicillin allergy—
ciprofloxacin, tetracycline, erythromycin)

Penicillinase producing N gonorrhoeae
ciprofloxacin

Tetracycline is the drug of choice for either chlamydia positive or chlamydia negative non-gonococcal salpingitis (details are given in the box at the end of the chapter). Since these two types of infection are often polymicrobial, metronidazole should also be given to eradicate any possible anaerobic infection. If the patient has severe pelvic inflammatory disease—for example, pelvic peritonitis—it may be necessary to start treatment intravenously before using oral regimens.

Gonococcal infection managed on an outpatient basis needs initial treatment with oral ampicillin/amoxycillin and probenecid. This is followed by a 14-day course of a tetracycline plus metronidazole. Patients may need to be hospitalised when intramuscular or intravenous therapy is used.

The US Centers for Disease Control recommend that a broad spectrum combination of antibiotics should be used from the outset to eradicate *N gonorrhoeae* and *C trachomatis* with or without anaerobes. (Full details are given in the box at the end of the chapter.) Thus examples of inpatient therapy would be intravenous doxycycline and cefoxitin or gentamicin and clindamycin and on an outpatient basis cefoxitin as an immediate dose followed by doxycycline by mouth for 10–14 days. This belt and braces approach is partly dictated by the fact that most patients with pelvic inflammatory disease in the USA are treated by private physicians, who often have no special knowledge of sexually acquired disease or access to microbiological support services.

For penicillinase producing strains of *N gonorrhoeae* ciprofloxacin is the drug of choice. If a patient with gonococcal salpingitis is allergic to penicillin then ciprofloxacin, tetracycline, or erythromycin may be used.

All sexual contacts of the patient should be traced, to prevent infection of others and reinfection of the patient. Seeing contacts in this way and taking specimens for microbiological tests also help in identifying likely causative organisms which may have been missed in the female partner.

Local complications: vulva

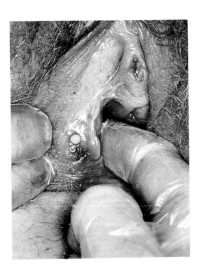

Bartholinitis or Bartholin's abscess is an uncommon complication of gonorrhoea. The patient may present with labial pain and swelling and sometimes difficulty in walking. Early in the condition pus may be visible or may be massaged out of the duct. Once an abscess has formed, however, a fluctuant mass will be felt. Specimens of pus should be collected from the duct (if draining), cervix, and urethra for microscopy and culture to isolate the gonococcus. *C trachomatis* should also be looked for since it may coexist with *N gonorrhoeae*. If *N gonorrhoeae* is identified and the duct is draining without an abscess having formed the patient should be treated with one intramuscular dose of procaine penicillin (2·4 MU), or oral ampicillin or amoxycillin 3 g followed by ampicillin/amoxycillin 500 mg four times a day for five to seven days. Probenicid should be given in association with penicillin. An abscess will not resolve adequately on antibiotics alone and marsupialisation is necessary to avoid further abscess formation. Sexual contacts should be investigated and urethral tests performed since, as with pelvic inflammatory disease, these often help in identifying the aetiological agent and preventing spread of the disease and reinfection.

Local complications: epididymis and testis

Differential diagnoses—epididymo-orchitis

- Testicular torsion
- Neoplasm
- Urinary tract infection
- Tubercle
- Viral infection

Epididymitis and orchitis due to a sexually transmitted agent are now rare. Patients with either condition or a combination (epididymo-orchitis) may also have a urethral discharge, but this is not invariable. A diagnosis of testicular torsion, urinary tract infection, neoplasm, or tubercle and viral infections affecting the testes (mumps, coxsackie, etc) should not be overlooked.

If gonorrhoea is confirmed by microscopy or culture of a sample of urethral discharge the usual treatment regimen of an initial dose of intramuscular or oral penicillin followed by oral ampicillin/amoxycillin and probenecid for seven days should be given. Non-gonococcal infections should be treated with tetracycline 500 mg four times a day or doxycycline 100 mg orally twice a day for two weeks. A scrotal support should be worn and in severe cases bed rest is necessary. Sexual contacts should be seen and investigated for chlamydia and gonorrhoea.

Local complications: prostate

Symptoms of prostatitis

Acute
Pyrexia ± rigors
Dysuria
Frequency
Urgency
Perianal pain

Chronic
Pain (suprapubic, perineal, low back, scrotal,
   thighs, penile tip, on ejaculation)
Dysuria
Frequency/nocturia
Urgency
Haematuria
Haemospermia
Low libido, impotence
Depression

Minocycline 100 mg twice a day for 2 weeks

Doxycycline 100 mg a day for 2–3 weeks

Erythromycin 250 mg four times a day for 3–4 weeks

Tetracycline 250 mg four times a day for 3–4 weeks

Ciprofloxacin 500 mg twice a day for 4–12 weeks

Prostatitis may be associated with gonococcal and non-gonococcal infections as well as with a urinary tract infection. Chronic prostatitis is more common than acute prostatitis. Though rare, prostatitis associated with gonorrhoea is usually acute. In acute disease frequency of micturition, dysuria, urgency, and fever are more common symptoms than pain. In chronic prostatitis pain is the most troublesome symptom; it may be suprapubic, perianal, lumbar, or scrotal; affect the thighs or tip of the penis; or be noticed only on ejaculation. Dysuria, frequency of micturition, haemospermia, low libido, impotence, or depression may also occur.

An accurate clinical history, thorough physical examination, and microbiological tests are all important in establishing a diagnosis. The prostate is only rarely tender and enlarged on rectal examination, and this is usually found in association with acute rather than chronic prostatitis. To obtain a specimen of prostatic secretion for microscopy and culture the prostate needs to be massaged. This procedure can precipitate an epididymitis in the presence of a posterior urethritis or cystitis and should not be carried out unless the second of the two glass urine test is clear.

The method used to obtain a specimen of prostatic fluid varies from straightforward massage to the Stamey technique of collecting urine both before and after the massage to differentiate between prostatitis, cystitis, and urethritis. More than 10 leucocytes per high power field ($\times 40$ magnification) or clumping of the cells, or both, in the prostatic secretion will indicate prostatitis. Further investigations of the urinary tract are indicated if a urinary tract infection is discovered.

If no organisms are identified on microscopy or culture of the prostatic fluid a broad spectrum antibiotic which is lipid soluble and so diffuses into the prostate should be given—for example, minocycline, doxycycline, or erythromycin. Tetracycline may be given, but it is less effective as it does not penetrate the prostate well. Finally, ciprofloxacin can be used in chronic bacterial prostatitis.

Occasionally patients may present with or develop two rare but serious complications affecting multiple sites.

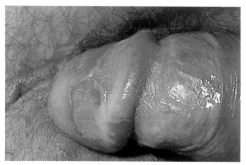

Circinate balanitis.

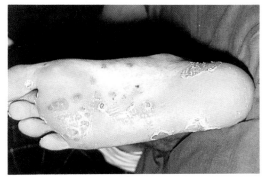

Keratoderma blenorrhagica.

Disseminated gonococcal infection

- Admit to hospital
- Give high doses of penicillin
- Trace all sexual contacts

Reiter's disease

Reiter's disease, which is a seronegative polyarthropathy occurring as a rare (0·5–1%) complication of non-gonococcal urethritis, affects mainly men. *C trachomatis, Shigella, Salmonella* and *Yersinia* have also been implicated in the aetiology of this condition. Conjunctivitis may also occur with the urethritis and arthritis but it is not an essential feature of the condition. The leg joints, particularly knees, ankles and feet, are those most commonly affected. Other manifestations are mucous membrane lesions of the mouth and penis (circinate balanitis), keratodermia blenorrhagica of the feet and hands, onycholysis and ridging of the nails, and, rarely, pericarditis, partial heart block, aortic incompetence, peripheral neuropathy, and meningoencephalitis. An accurate clinical history is essential to exclude other arthropathies, such as rheumatoid arthritis and ankylosing spondylitis and those occurring with psoriasis, Crohn's disease, and ulcerative colitis.

Non-steroidal anti-inflammatory agents are given in mild cases—for example, indomethacin 25 mg three times a day. Bed rest, but not total immobilisation, is recommended during the active phase of the disease. Systemic steroids should be reserved for seriously ill patients or for those with complications such as pericarditis and uveitis. A concurrent non-gonococcal urethritis should be treated with tetracycline. The prognosis of Reiter's disease is extremely variable and relapses do occur.

Disseminated gonococcal infection

Disseminated gonococcal infection is a rare complication of gonorrhoea and affects women more often than men. The common symptoms are pain in the joints (wrists, knees, elbows, ankles, or small joints of the hand), tenosynovitis, and rash. The initial erythematous macular papular lesions develop into frank vesicles and pustules; they appear as crops on the trunk and arms and legs and often in association with a fever. Occasionally endocarditis, myocarditis, pericarditis, and meningitis may occur. Gonococci are often isolated from the genital tract and occasionally from blood and joint fluid but rarely from skin lesions. Patients need to be admitted to hospital and treated with high doses of penicillin. All sexual contacts must be traced.

Infections in other sites

Rectum—The rectum may be affected in several sexually transmitted conditions (gonorrhoea, chlamydia, non-gonococcal infections, genital herpes and warts, syphilis, *Entamoeba histolytica, Giardia lamblia,* and trauma). Only gonorrhoea is considered in this chapter. Rectal gonorrhoea is often symptomless and illustrates the need for contact tracing and regular check ups for homosexuals who are having casual sexual encounters. Symptoms, when they occur, are anal discomfort and pain, painful defecation, and a blood stained or purulent rectal discharge. Diagnosis is by microscopy and culture. Microscopy is incorrect in half of all cases since it is difficult to identify gonococci in the presence of many other organisms in the rectum. Cultures must always be performed if rectal gonorrhoea is suspected. Treatment and follow up of rectal gonorrhoea are the same as those for uncomplicated urethral or cervical infections.

Throat—Even though still uncommon, oropharyngeal gonorrhoea is being seen more often and may be asymptomatic. Patients admitting to orogenital contact will have throat swabs taken in a clinic in an attempt to isolate *N gonorrhoeae*. Patients with infection of the throat but no other site may also infect their partner's urethra during fellatio. Diagnosis is by culture; microscopy is useless owing to the presence of mixed organisms, particularly commensal neisseriae. In patients with pharyngeal infection ciprofloxacin 500 mg or ceftriaxone 250 mg orally are recommended treatments.

Treatment of acute pelvic inflammatory disease

Outpatient		Hospital	
Chlamydia positive or chlamydia negative, non-gonococcal	Gonococcal	Chlamydia positive or chlamydia negative, non-gonococcal	Gonococcal

Bed rest

Tetracycline 500 mg four times a day for 14 days + Metronidazole 400 mg twice daily for 14 days or Doxycycline 100 mg twice daily for 14 days + Metronidazole 400 mg twice daily for 14 days	Ampicillin/amoxycillin 3 g orally +probenicid 1 g **Followed by** Doxycycline 100 mg twice daily for 14 days + Metronidazole 400 mg twice daily for 14 days	Tetracycline or doxycycline + Metronidazole as for outpatient treatment or Tetracycline or doxycycline + Metronidazole intravenously until clinical improvement ↓ Continue orally as for outpatient treatment	Procaine penicillin intramuscularly or ampicillin/amoxycillin intravenously ↓ **Until clinical improvement** Doxycycline 100 mg twice daily for 14 days + Metronidazole 400 mg twice daily for 14 days

1 Penicillinase producing *N gonorrhoeae*	Ciprofloxacin 500 mg followed by a tetracycline +metronidazole as above
2 Patients allergic to penicillin, with gonococcal pelvic inflammatory disease	Ciprofloxacin 500 mg (unless pregnant) Tetracycline 500 mg four times a day for 14 days + Metronidazole for 14 days Doxycycline 100 mg twice daily for 14 days + Metronidazole for 14 days Erythromycin stearate 500 mg four times a day for 14 days

---

Centres for Disease Control (CDC) guidelines for treatment of pelvic inflammatory disease (1998)

Outpatient regimens

Regimen A

Ofloxacin 400 mg orally twice a day for 14 days
PLUS
Metronidazole 500 mg orally twice a day for 14 days

Regimen B

Ceftriaone 250 mg IM once
OR
Cefoxitin 2 g IM plus **probenecid** 1 g orally in a single dose concurrently once
OR
Other parental third-generation **cephalosporin** (eg **ceftizoxime** or **cefotaxime**)
PLUS
Doxycycline 100 mg orally twice a day for 14 days. (Include this regimen with one of the above regimens)

Inpatient regimens

One of the alternatives A and B given for at least 48 hours after the patient demonstrates substantial clinical improvement, after which, consider switch to oral therapy

Parenteral Regimen A

Cefotetan 2 g IV every 12 hours
OR
Cefoxitin 2 g IV every 6 hours
PLUS
Doxycycline 100 mg IV or orally every 12 hours

OR

Parenteral Regimen B

Clindamycin 900 mg IV every 8 hours
PLUS
Gentamicin loading dose IV or IM (2 mg/kg of body weight), followed by a maintenance dose (1.5 mg/kg) every 8 hours. Single daily dosing may be substituted

The illustration of Bartholin's abscess is reproduced from King A, Nicol C, Rodin P. *Venereal Diseases*, published by Baillière Tindall.

GENITAL ULCERATION

Multiple and painful	Solitary and painful
Multiple and painless	Solitary and painless

Genital ulceration (or erosion) is a common symptom in both sexes and is often due to a sexually transmitted agent. Particular points that need to be elicited from the patient to aid diagnosis are the number of ulcers, the time they have been present, the degree of discomfort they cause and the relation of their appearance to sexual intercourse, trauma, and lesions elsewhere. Most ulcers or erosions are either multiple and painful or solitary and painless.

Multiple painful ulcers

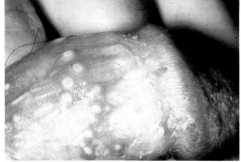

Primary herpes

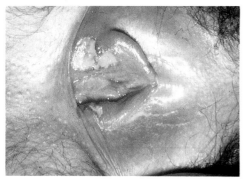

Behçet's disease

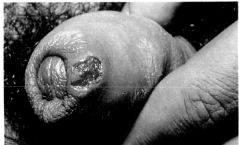

Chancroid

Multiple ulcers, particularly if painful, are at present in the United Kingdom most commonly due to an infection with herpes simplex virus. If this is the patient's first attack the ulcers occur within one to two weeks of exposure to infection. The inguinal lymph nodes are enlarged, discrete, and usually painful. There may be systemic illness including fever, headache, and myalgia. A recurrent attack is unlikely to bear any relation to sexual intercourse; it is sometimes preceded by prodromal symptoms and the patient often volunteers the diagnosis (see next chapter). Herpes zoster rarely gives rise to genital ulceration.

Other causes of painful multiple ulcers are Behçet's disease and, rarely in the United Kingdom, chancroid caused by *Haemophilus ducreyi*. Behçet's disease is usually associated with oral ulcers and chancroid is invariably contracted abroad or from a sexual partner who has recently returned from abroad. Chancroid has an extremely short incubation period of two to five days. Scabies may also rarely present as multiple, itching, painful, secondarily infected ulcerated papules produced by scratching.

Patients with non-gonococcal, gonococcal, trichomonal, and candidal infections may have multiple painful erosive lesions on the penis and vulva, sometimes with fissuring. Balanitis and vulvitis may also be found in infections with β haemolytic streptococci and Vincent's organisms. Similar lesions may occur as part of the Stevens-Johnson or Reiter's syndrome, or be due to erythema multiforme, dermatitis, psoriasis and lichen planus, impetigo, furuncles, folliculitis, and drug eruptions.

Solitary painless ulcers

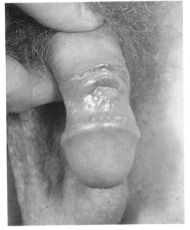
Primary syphilis

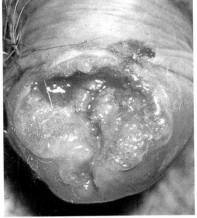
Carcinoma of penis

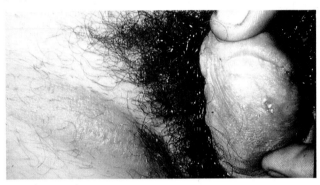
Lymphogranuloma venereum

The commonest cause of painless genital ulceration is primary syphilis. The incubation period is usually 21 days but the lesions may appear from nine to 90 days after sexual intercourse with an infected partner. Inguinal lymph nodes are moderately enlarged, painless, and discrete. Other stages of syphilis may also result in genital ulceration. Ulcers of the secondary stage, evident as eroded papules or mucous patches, will be multiple but painless, whereas a gumma is usually solitary, painless, and a tertiary manifestation. Other causes of solitary painless ulcers are carcinoma, circinate balanitis, balanitis xerotica obliterans, lymphogranuloma venereum, and granuloma inguinale. Self inflicted trauma or dermatitis artefacta may give rise to large solitary ulcerated areas which are suprisingly painless. More traumatic lesions of the penis, anus, and rectum usually result from sadomasochistic practices.

Diagnosis

Causes of genital ulceration and erosions

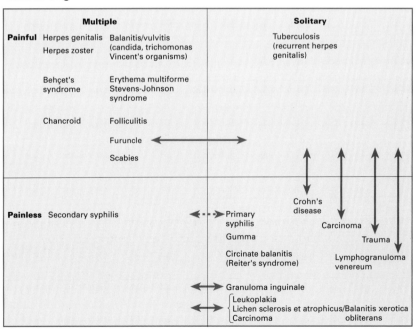

	Multiple		Solitary	
Painful	Herpes genitalis Herpes zoster	Balanitis/vulvitis (candida, trichomonas Vincent's organisms)	Tuberculosis (recurrent herpes genitalis)	
	Behçet's syndrome	Erythema multiforme Stevens-Johnson syndrome		
	Chancroid	Folliculitis		
		Furuncle		
		Scabies		
Painless	Secondary syphilis	Primary syphilis Gumma	Crohn's disease Carcinoma	
		Circinate balanitis (Reiter's syndrome)	Trauma Lymphogranuloma venereum	
		Granuloma inguinale		
		Leukoplakia Lichen sclerosis et atrophicus/Balanitis xerotica Carcinoma	obliterans	

The two commonest causes of genital ulceration in the United Kingdom are herpes and syphilis. These often look different on macroscopic examination, but the naked eye should not be relied on to differentiate between them or confirm the diagnosis. Herpes is diagnosed by culture of the virus. To exclude primary or secondary syphilis, three separate specimens of serum from the ulcer(s) should be examined by dark ground microscopy initially and on three consecutive days. Serological tests for syphilis are not always positive when primary syphilitic lesions are present; the tests do not become positive for about three to four weeks after infection, whereas a primary lesion or chancre may be evident as soon as nine to ten days after exposure (see Chapter 15).

If the ulceration is due to circinate balanitis, scabies, or Behçet's syndrome, other extragenital lesions may usually be found. The three tropical conditions of chancroid, lymphogranuloma venereum, and granuloma inguinale require special culture facilities. In addition to investigating the cause of the presenting symptom of genital ulceration, tests must be carried out to exclude other concurrent sexually transmitted diseases contracted at the same time and to determine the underlying cause of the ulcers or erosions.

GENITAL HERPES

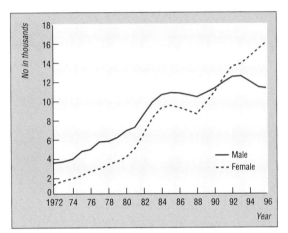

Cases of genital herpes seen in GUM clinics: England

Problems associated with genital herpes

- Increasing

- No curative treatment

- Recurrent

- Breakdown of relationships/
  psychosexual problems/depression
- Neonatal infections

Genital infection with herpes simplex virus poses five problems. It is increasing, it is an unpleasant disease with no cure, and it is recurrent, the last two of which may lead to breakdown of relationships, psychosexual problems, and depression; and, finally, it may cause neonatal and possibly fetal infections.

The latest figures (1996) show that 27 496 cases of genital herpes were seen in departments of genitourinary medicine in England. The number of cases has levelled off in recent years. These figures make it the fourth most common sexually transmitted disease. Certainly, more cases exist than are diagnosed in departments of genitourinary medicine and these will be managed in general practice or by gynaecologists and dermatologists. In the United States it is estimated that 22% of people age 12 years or older have herpes simplex type 2 (HSV2) antibodies corresponding to 45 million infected individuals.

The virus

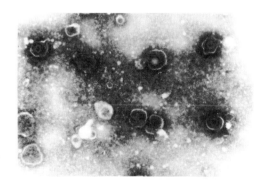

Herpes simplex virus is a double stranded DNA virus which can be classified into types 1 and 2. Both types can cause genital infection even though type 1 usually causes lesions of the face, lips, and eyes. The prevalence of type 1 infection varies inversely with socioeconomic state. Type 1 and type 2 antibodies are thought to offer some cross protection, and the reduction in type 1 infection and antibody development during childhood in developed countries may be a factor in the increase in genital herpes in such countries.

The virus is transmitted by sexual intercourse or other physical contact. Orogenital contact with a partner with type 1 labial lesions may result in genital herpes. The illness may range from being entirely asymptomatic to being a severe systemic and mucocutaneous disease.

Primary infections

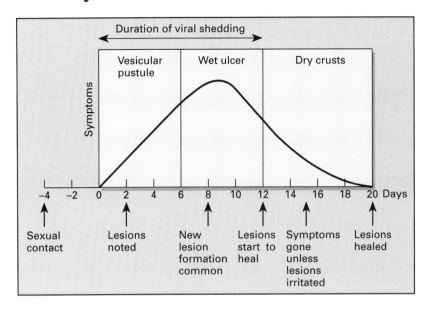

A first attack (primary herpes) of genital herpes usually presents with multiple painful genital ulcers after a short incubation period of under seven days. The amount of pain experienced by the patient varies depending on the number and site of the lesions. All the skin lesions, whether on the genitals themselves or on adjacent areas (buttocks, thighs, anus), evolve in the same way—starting with erythema, progressing to vesicles then ulcers, and finishing with crusting. The separate lesions often coalesce into substantial areas of shallow ulceration. These local lesions and viral shedding last about 12 days, with healing taking a further week, so that the whole illness may last for three weeks. In most primary attacks in women both the vulva and the cervix are affected (80–90% of cases). Nevertheless, single sites may be affected so that cervical lesions may be present without vulval lesions and vice versa.

Inguinal lymphadenopathy occurs in most primary cases and about half of these patients actually complain of pain in the groin. Anorectal herpes can cause pain, discharge, and constipation. About one third of patients may have vague constitutional symptoms of fever and malaise and about 10% headache, photophobia, and viral meningitis. Retention of urine is a very rare symptom and in most instances is due to the patient's understandable reluctance to pass urine over already painful lesions; occasionally it is due to the virus affecting the sacral autonomic plexus, with a resulting meningomyelitis.

Site	Symptoms					
	Pain	Dysuria	Retention	Constipation	Discharge	None
Penis (glans, coronal sulcus and shaft)	+					±
Urethra (male)	++	+	+		+	+
Anus/rectum	+		±	+	+	+
Buttocks/thighs/ scrotum	+					
Vulva/urethra	++	+	±		±	±
Vagina	+				+	±
Cervix	+				++	+

Recurrent infections

Recurrent infections are less severe and are not due to reinfection. Patients offer a variety of precipitating causes for their recurrences such as stress, sexual intercourse, menstruation, and climatic changes. Epidemiological data suggest that the mean time interval between initial and recurrent infection is about 120 days (range 25–360 days). The rate of recurrence, however, is to some extent dependent on viral type. Patients with HSV 2 tend to suffer recurrences earlier after the primary infection and then more frequently than those with type 1 infection. Patients often notice prodromal symptoms of local tingling and parasthesiae for 24–48 hours before the onset of lesions. The recurrent infection is not only milder but also shorter than the initial attack. There are fewer, but identical, lesions which heal more rapidly than previously. Systemic manifestations are rare.

Patients with both initial and recurrent attacks may be asymptomatic, unaware that they have infection or have minor complaints which are not attributed to herpes. Some studies suggest that up to 50% of patients fall into these groups. This raises considerable problems not only for the patient but also in relation to control of the disease within the community.

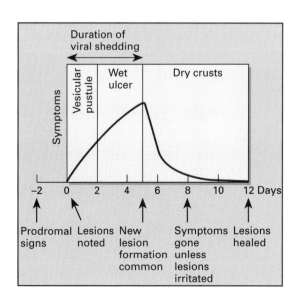

The diagnosis

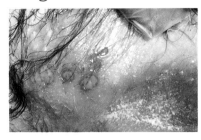

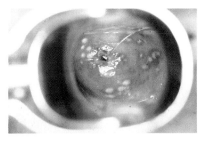

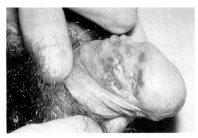

Lesions on vulva, cervix, and penis.

The clinical history and examination usually give the doctor a good idea of the eventual diagnosis. Nevertheless, the ulceration has to be differentiated from syphilis by dark ground microscopy. Other sexually transmitted diseases such as gonorrhoea, chlamydial infections, and trichomoniasis, which could have been contracted at the same time, must be excluded by full microbiological tests. Serological tests for syphilis should be taken as a base line.

The cervix may be ulcerated, frankly necrotic, or appear normal. The definitive diagnosis of genital herpes can be made only by viral culture and isolation of the organism. Newer immunoassays are becoming increasingly available for diagnosis. They are not so sensitive as culture but have the advantage of speed and the ability to type the virus. Similarly, a homosexual patient who complains only of anal lesions should have tests carried out for herpes and other sexually transmitted conditions. Most patients with a primary attack of herpes will not tolerate the passing of a speculum or proctoscope and this may have to be delayed until symptoms have improved.

Material for culture should be taken with a sterile cotton wool swab which is rubbed over the lesions so that adequate serum is obtained. If only vesicles are present, one or two of them may need to be punctured to obtain the specimen. This should be placed in a viral transport medium, refrigerated at 4°C, and sent to the laboratory on the same day. Since herpes is a chronic and incurable infection the diagnosis must always be confirmed by culture. It is unfair to the patient as well as to his or her sexual contacts to make such a diagnosis on clinical grounds. These may mislead, and a wrong diagnosis may create unnecessary anxiety for more than one person.

Routine management

- Bathe lesions in warm saline
- Analgesics
- Treat secondary infections
- Admit to hospital if:
  Uncontrollable pain
  Urinary retention
  ? Meningitis

The treatment of genital herpes still remains unsatisfactory and no cure is yet available. The conservative palliative approach should be the basis of management. To some extent pain may be alleviated by bathing the lesions in warm saline (a teaspoon of domestic salt added to 0·5 l of warm tap water); this also helps to keep the lesions clean. If the lesions are particularly severe patients may be encouraged to sit in a warm bath to which salt has been added (three tablespoons). Patients often find that swishing the water around the lesions while sitting in the bath is soothing and that it is easier to pass urine. Pain may also be relieved by simple analgesics, and some patients find relief by the use of ice packs. Occasionally secondary infection occurs and should be treated with an appropriate antibiotic, preferably one that is non-treponemicidal and will, therefore, not mask syphilis. Some patients are so ill, usually during the initial attack, that they require admission to hospital. The indications for this are uncontrollable pain, urinary retention, and possible meningitis.

Antiviral agents and vaccines

Treatment
- Acyclovir, famciclovir, valaciclovir
- Do not use steroids

Acyclovir acts on a specific viral enzyme thus preventing viral replication. Studies using this drug in primary and recurrent attacks have shown that viral shedding, healing time, and duration of symptoms may be reduced but that the subsequent development of recurrences is not affected. Oral acyclovir is useful in primary attacks. It can be given in a dose of 200 mg orally, five times a day for five days in patients with particularly severe lesions. Acyclovir is of limited use if the lesions have been present for more than six days. Other agents such as famciclovir or valaciclovir can be used. Recurrences can only be prevented by continuous prophylactic use which is expensive. Usually prophylactic treatment is not indicated unless the patient has about six attacks per year. Treatment should be started at a dose of 200 mg four times a day or 400 mg twice a day. This dose can be reduced after eight weeks if the patient has had no recurrences. Famciclovir or valaciclovir can also be used as suppressive therapy.

Treatment should be stopped at one year and the frequency of recurrences assessed before giving further treatment. Acyclovir cream is of marginal benefit for the treatment of primary and recurrent episodes. No effective vaccine presently exists; those being developed still need to be tested by randomised controlled trials.

Counselling and other problems

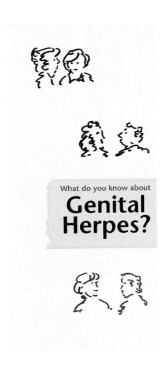

Genital herpes is an emotive disease, particularly since it is recurrent and may interfere with sexual intercourse. Patients often need a great deal of advice and emotional support and since the condition is incurable, it is important that doctors at least fulfil these two functions. Patients should be warned that they are infectious when lesions are present; they should therefore abstain from sexual intercourse once lesions are noted or sooner if prodromal symptoms are present. Since lesions are widespread, particularly in women, the sheath will not always stop contact with infected areas and is not therefore effective in preventing infection during an attack. Since asymptomatic infection and viral shedding can exist the regular use of condoms between overt attacks will need to be discussed with patients. Likewise patients should be reminded that other forms of intimacy and close bodily contact, apart from sexual intercourse, are not precluded. They often find it useful to talk to fellow sufferers, and SPHERE (previously the Herpes Association) is a self help group that patients find useful.

Two major concerns relating to genital herpes are the possible effects on the fetus and neonate and, in the long term, on the cervix. (The problems of in utero and neonatal infection are covered in a later chapter.)

Reproduced with permission from SmithKline Beecham.

The illustrations of the clinical course of primary and recurrent infections were reproduced by permission of Dr L Corey.

VIRAL HEPATITIS

IAN VD WELLER, RICHARD JC GILSON

Causes and epidemiology

	Typical incubation period	Transmission routes	Carrier state
Hepatitis A	4–6 weeks	Faecal–oral, sexual (homosexual)	None
Hepatitis B	12 weeks	Parenteral, percutaneous, perinatal, sexual (homosexual and heterosexual)	5% adults 90% infants
Hepatitis C	8 weeks	Parenteral, percutaneous, (particularly blood/blood products, if not screened, and injecting drug users), sexual/vertical(low risk)	60–70%
Hepatitis D	7 weeks	Parenteral (coinfection with acute hepatitis B or superinfection of hepatitis B carrier)	About 2% if coinfection, 70-80% if superinfection
Hepatitis E	3–6 weeks	Faecal-oral (in tropics)	None

Hepatitis is the characteristic feature of infection with several different viruses, referred to as hepatitis A to E, in approximately the order in which they were recognised. The clinical features of acute infection with these viruses are not readily distinguishable; all may cause an acute illness with jaundice, but commonly cause asymptomatic infection. Some cause chronic infection, which may progress to cirrhosis, end-stage liver disease and hepatocellular carcinoma. The most important sexually transmitted hepatitis virus is hepatitis B; high rates of transmission have been reported; it causes chronic liver disease, and it can be prevented by vaccination. Other viruses occasionally cause a hepatitis including cytomegalovirus and Epstein–Barr virus.

Hepatitis A is caused by a small RNA virus, which is excreted in the stools for up to 2 weeks before the onset of symptoms. Childhood infection, usually asymptomatic, is common, but with improving standards of hygiene in the developed world an increasing proportion of adults are still susceptible; only about 20% of young adults in London are immune. There is evidence for sexual transmission of hepatitis A among homosexual men, by oral–anal contact. Although sexual transmission probably contributes little to their overall risk of infection, outbreaks of hepatitis A in homosexual men have been reported. Except in rare cases of fulminant disease, full recovery after hepatitis A occurs; there is no carrier state and immunity is lifelong.

Hepatitis B is caused by a small DNA virus, detectable in serum several weeks before the acute illness. Those with persistent infection, hepatitis B carriers, represent the main pool of infectious individuals. In regions with a high carrier rate, for example tropical Africa and South East Asia, 8–20% of the population carry the virus. Peak incidence occurs during the perinatal period, during early childhood and adolescence. In regions with a low carrier rate, such as the UK, only about 1 in 1000 of the population carry the virus, but certain groups are at high risk of infection including homosexual men and injecting drug users. Risk factors are multiple casual sexual partners, anal intercourse, and sharing of injecting equipment. Up to 5% of homosexual men and injecting drug users attending STD clinics in the UK are carriers and 25–50% are immune due to previous infection.

Hepatitis D is caused by a defective RNA virus which needs hepatitis B virus to produce infection. Transmitted with hepatitis B virus, it causes a dual acute infection, which usually resolves. More

Groups at risk of infection with hepatitis B

Endemic areas

Whole population (peak incidence as neonate/early childhood and adolescence)

Low-endemicity areas (for example, UK)

- Neonates of carrier mothers
- Homosexual men
- Prostitutes
- Injecting drug users
- Sexual contact(s) of acute cases and carriers
- Household contacts of HBeAg-positive carriers
- Certain patients, laboratory and medical staff exposed to blood or blood products or in closed institutions

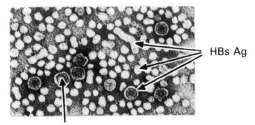

HBs Ag

HBc – contains DNA, DNA polymerase and e antigen (also free in serum)

importantly, it can occur as a superinfection in carriers of hepatitis B virus, causing an intercurrent, and potentially severe hepatitis. Chronic superinfection occurs in up to 90% with worsening of chronic liver disease. Hepatitis D is more common in injecting drug users and haemophiliacs. Infection in homosexual men is rare in the UK but has been reported in 14% of carriers of hepatitis B virus elsewhere.

Hepatitis C. Another type of viral hepatitis, termed non-A, non-B hepatitis, was recognised soon after specific tests for hepatitis A and hepatitis B were developed. Eventually, in 1989, hepatitis C virus was identified, and commercial antibody assays became available in 1990–91. Over 90% of non-A, non-B hepatitis cases are caused by hepatitis C virus. The principal route of transmission is by percutaneous inoculation, blood, and blood products. In developed countries individuals most at risk are those who have received multiple blood transfusions or blood products prior to the introduction of blood donor screening (September 1991 in the UK) and those with any history of injecting drug use. Hepatitis C accounts for 15–30% of cases of sporadic acute hepatitis. In 25–30% of patients there is no history of parenteral exposure suggesting transmission by person to person or sexual contact. In studies of homosexual men, the prevalence of hepatitis C, typically about 1%, is much lower than that of hepatitis B or HIV, although this may still be higher than heterosexual controls. Studies of sexual partners (homosexual and heterosexual) of patients with hepatitis C have found a low prevalence of infection. These data are consistent with a low rate of transmission of hepatitis C by sexual contact.

Hepatitis E, caused by a small RNA virus, is the principal cause of the enterically transmitted form of non-A, non-B hepatitis. Spread by the faecal–oral route, hepatitis E virus causes waterborne epidemics in South East and Central Asia, Africa and North America. It has an incubation period similar to that of hepatitis A and no carrier state has been reported. It is associated with a high mortality during pregnancy; sexual transmission has not been implicated.

Hepatitis F has yet to be identified but is being sought as a possible cause of fulminant hepatitis, particularly in those cases where hepatitis A, B, and C virus infections appear not to be responsible.

Hepatitis G virus has recently been identified from material from cases of non-A, non-B, non-C hepatitis. Structurally it is closely related to hepatitis C. It appears to be transmitted in blood or blood products and is often associated with hepatitis C coinfection. However, there remains much uncertainty as to how often it is associated with liver disease, either acute or chronic; in most cases of infection there is no evidence of inflammatory liver disease, and it is not a cause of fulminant hepatitis.

History and examination

It is important to ask about sexual orientation and contacts and whether the partner has symptoms of hepatitis. Most cases of acute hepatitis diagnosed in STD clinics occur in homosexual men and are due to hepatitis A or B viruses. Any history of travel, injecting drug use, tattoos, recent transfusion, or other percutaneous exposure should be obtained. Hepatotoxins such as alcohol and drugs should be excluded as a cause of hepatitis. The clinical illness begins with non-specific symptoms such as fever, headache, and fatigue, and jaundice follows. Symptoms and signs of other concurrent sexually transmitted diseases should be looked for. More than half of acute infections are subclinical. There are no major differences in the clinical features of the acute illness caused by any of the hepatitis viruses.

Laboratory tests

Routine liver function tests are unhelpful in identifying the responsible virus. They may help to distinguish between hepatitis and cholestasis due to extrahepatic or intrahepatic lesions, but prolonged cholestasis occurs occasionally with acute viral hepatitis. Tests of synthetic function such as prothrombin time and serum albumin are useful in assessing the severity of the hepatitis.

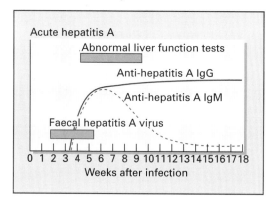

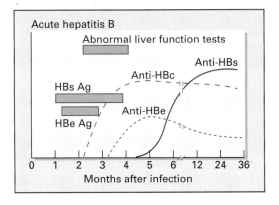

Specific serological tests

Hepatitis A, Epstein–Barr virus and cytomegalovirus infections are best diagnosed by tests for specific serum IgM antibodies, which persist for a short time and indicate recent infection. IgG antibodies appear more slowly but persist for many years.

Early in acute hepatitis B, hepatitis B surface (HBsAg) and hepatitis B e antigens (HBeAg) appear in the serum. Rarely, HBsAg may disappear before the onset of clinical symptoms. Anti-HBc becomes detectable during the acute illness. If an assay for anti-HBcIgM is strongly reactive this helps to distinguish between an acute infection and a carrier. In a resolving infection, HBeAg soon becomes undetectable with the appearance of anti-HBe. Anti-HBs, the only antibody indicative of immunity, becomes detectable in serum after HBsAg has cleared, although there may be an interval of weeks or months when neither HBsAg nor anti-HBs are detectable. If HBsAg remains detectable for more than 6 months the patient has, by the usual definition, become a hepatitis B virus carrier.

Hepatitis C infection is diagnosed by the detection of antibodies or viral nucleic acid. The first generation of assays detected antibody only to a recombinant protein derived from the non-structural, NS4 region. Subsequent assays have been made more sensitive and specific by the use of a larger NS3/NS4 peptide (C200, a putative helicase) and the addition of recombinant antigens from the core region (C22) and NS5 (an RNA-dependent RNA polymerase). Supplementary assays employing different formats enable responses to individual antigens to be detected and scored; unequivocal reactivity to at least two antigens are interpreted as confirmation. Anti-HCV assays are of limited value in diagnosing acute infection, seroconversion being delayed by 4–12 weeks. HCV-RNA can be detected by polymerase chain reaction or signal amplification assays, which enables earlier diagnosis of acute infection. HCV antibodies are not neutralising; most patients found to have HCV antibodies on screening are viral carriers, which can be confirmed by HCV-RNA detection.

Hepatitis D is diagnosed by antibody assays for anti-HDV in HBsAg-positive patients. Hepatitis E virus infection can be diagnosed by antibody assays. Detectable antibodies may be lost following recovery from infection. Assays for HGV are available for research purposes.

In all patients with hepatitis that may have been acquired sexually, other sexually transmitted diseases should be excluded by taking appropriate specimens for microscopy and culture from exposed sites and performing serological tests for syphilis.

Complications

Fulminant hepatitis is a rare complication occurring in less than 1% of patients with all types of acute viral hepatitis. The severity of acute hepatitis A increases with age and pre-existing liver disease (including chronic hepatitis B or C). As the general population prevalence of immunity to hepatitis A falls, there is concern that more symptomatic and severe cases will be seen.

Up to 90% of neonates infected with hepatitis B become chronic carriers, the proportion falling rapidly to age 5–6. Thereafter, about 5% of patients with acute hepatitis B become carriers, less if the acute infection was symptomatic, more if the patient is immunosuppressed. Chronic carriers initially have high levels of viral replication with complete virus particles and HBeAg detectable in the serum. These carriers are of high infectivity. Liver biopsy is the most reliable way of assessing the activity of the inflammatory liver disease, and the presence of fibrosis.

Chronic hepatitis B with little inflammatory liver disease activity (chronic persistent hepatitis) is usually benign. Some patients do, however, develop more severe disease (chronic active hepatitis), particularly those in whom HBeAg to anti-HBe seroconversion is delayed. Progression to cirrhosis and end-stage liver disease may follow. Cirrhosis is associated with a greatly increased risk of primary hepatocellular carcinoma. Most patients who have lost detectable serum HBeAg, and seroconverted to anti-HBe, have normal liver

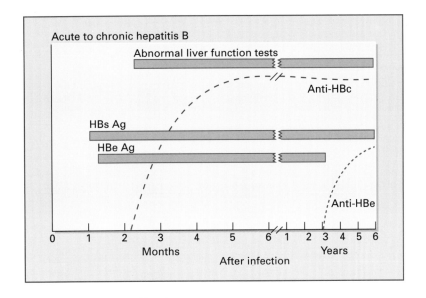

Acute to chronic hepatitis B

Interactions between infection with HIV and hepatitis B virus

Epidemiology
↓ Incidence of hepatitis B because of changing sexual behaviour

Clinical effects
? Incidence of fulminant hepatitis reduced
↑ Infectivity of HBV carriers
↓ Hepatic inflammatory activity
↓ Response rate to vaccine
↑ Loss of natural and vaccine-induced antibodies
↓ Response to antiviral treatment
? Effect on risk of cirrhosis and hepatocellular carcinoma unknown

transaminase levels and liver histology. These patients are at low risk of serious sequelae. Some patients with anti-HBe, carry viruses with mutations in the hepatitis B precore gene sequence. These patients are more likely to have detectable viraemia and are therefore more likely to transmit infection. They may also be at increased risk of serious liver disease.

Concomitant infection with hepatitis B and HIV is common. Interactions between these two infections include an increased rate of progression to the HBV carrier state following acute infection, higher HBV replication rate, and reduced spontaneous loss of HBeAg. The effect on the epidemiology of HBV infection would be to increase the pool of infectious carriers. Although the activity of HBV-associated inflammatory liver disease may be reduced in patients with HIV infection, cases of rapidly progressive liver disease have also been reported; in most cohort studies to date, mortality is still largely determined by other HIV-related complications.

Acute infection with hepatitis C virus is usually mild but becomes chronic in an estimated 60–70% of cases; the exact proportion is uncertain, and may depend on the route of transmission. The clinical course of chronic hepatitis C is similar to that of chronic hepatitis B. The proportion developing clinically significant liver disease is uncertain (estimate 10–30%), but rarely occurs within 10 years of infection. HIV coinfection may accelerate the progression of HCV-related chronic liver disease. Those who do not develop chronic infection may lose detectable antibodies.

Management

Indications for admission to hospital with acute hepatitis

Complications
Symptoms and signs of acute liver failure (signs of hepatic encephalopathy)

Doubts about diagnosis
Possible extrahepatic cause for jaundice

Social factors
Patient living alone

Acute viral hepatitis is usually self limiting and management is largely supportive. Most patients can be managed as outpatients, but acute liver failure and its complications demand urgent hospital admission.

In uncomplicated cases a low fat, high energy diet is more palatable and bed rest advisable during the early phase of the illness. Alcohol should be avoided until liver function tests are normal.

In chronic hepatitis, management is largely supportive; however antiviral treatment with alfa interferon is now an option for both hepatitis B and C. Treatment of hepatitis B is limited by the response rate (25–50% loss of HBeAg depending upon pretreatment characteristics), adverse effects, and cost. Predictors of response include a low serum HBV DNA concentration, high transaminase levels, and more active disease on liver biopsy, but these patients are also more likely to seroconvert spontaneously to anti-HBe. Treatment is not indicated for carriers with anti-HBe and normal biochemical and histological findings, who should be reassured. Alcohol may hasten the progression of chronic liver disease. There is much interest in new treatments for hepatitis B. Nucleoside analogues including lamivudine, famciclovir and adefovir are in clinical trial; all show activity in suppressing HBV replication. Other approaches, including immunotherapy, are also being investigated.

Chronic hepatitis C may also respond to alfa interferon therapy. Response is also limited (50% lose detectable HCV-RNA and normalise liver transaminases), but half of responders relapse quickly. Recommended treatment duration is longer than for hepatitis B (6–12 months versus 3–4 months) but the dose is lower, so that adverse effects are reduced. Some predictors of a better response (shorter duration of infection, low level of viraemia and certain genotypes) have been reported. Combination treatment with agents such as ribavirin may improve the sustained response rate.

Prevention

Prevention of hepatitis as a sexually transmitted disease

- Contact tracing

- Counselling of HBeAg-positive carriers

- Passive immunisation
  Hepatitis A—normal human immunoglobulin
  Hepatitis B—hepatitis B immunoglobulin (HBIg)

- Active immunisation—vaccine

- Safer sex/barrier contraception
  hepatitis C (no vaccine available)
  hepatitis A (avoid oral–anal exposure)

Because of the lack of effective treatment, prevention is paramount in the control of viral hepatitis.

The spread of hepatitis A can be controlled by applying simple hygienic precautions. Recent sexual contacts can be protected by passive immunisation with human normal immunoglobulin. Inactivated hepatitis A vaccines are available which provide protection after only one dose. With a booster dose at 6–12 months long-term immunity (> 10 years) is expected. It is recommended for the protection of long-term or frequent foreign travellers. Immunisation of homosexual men whose sexual behaviour places them at risk has been recommended, but those at risk are not well defined. Routine prophylaxis of all homosexual men is not currently recommended.

Hepatitis B transmission to carers and other contacts can be limited by careful handling of blood, blood-contaminated material, and instruments. However those at risk should be given specific prophylaxis. Sexual contacts of patients with acute hepatitis B should be traced and offered vaccine and, if seen within about 48 hours of an isolated contact, hepatitis B immunoglobulin as passive prophylaxis. Tracing of hepatitis B contacts is also important to identify HBV-infected individuals, usually HBeAg-positive carriers, who may have been the source of infection. These patients can then be counselled about their infectivity and protection of other non-immune sexual contacts can be provided.

The standard HBsAg vaccines contain hepatitis B S-protein, manufactured by recombinant DNA technology in yeast cell cultures, although in some parts of the world plasma-derived vaccines are still used. They are safe and protect over 90% of young immunocompetent vaccinees for at least 5 years. New vaccines containing preS1 and preS2 proteins, in addition, are being tested and may prove useful in overcoming non-response to the standard vaccines.

In low prevalence countries, such as the UK, the hepatitis B vaccine policy is to target those most at risk, while in many other countries universal immunisation of infants or adolescents (or both initially) is being implemented. Savings can be made by pretesting for HBV markers those in high prevalence groups, such as homosexual men, and by not screening others, such as health-care staff. Postvaccine testing to confirm response (or current infection if not prescreened) is advised. Non-responders, or poor responders may benefit from a further dose of vaccine. The need for routine booster doses is debated. Although unlikely to be cost effective at a population level, individuals may still be given a single booster dose at 5-year intervals, or longer in those with a vigorous postvaccine antibody response.

ACQUIRED IMMUNODEFICENCY SYNDROME

IAN G WILLIAMS, IAN WELLER

Definition

AIDS is defined as an illness characterised by one or more indicator diseases. In the absence of another cause of immune deficiency and without laboratory evidence of HIV infection (if the patient has not been tested or the results are inconclusive), certain diseases when definitely diagnosed are indicative of AIDS. Regardless of the presence of other causes of immune deficiency, if there is laboratory evidence of HIV infection other indicator diseases that require a definitive, or in some cases only a presumptive, diagnosis also constitute a diagnosis of AIDS.

In 1993 the Centres for Disease Control in the USA extended the definition of AIDS to include all persons who are severely immunosuppressed (a CD4 count $< 200 \times 10^6/l$) irrespective of the presence or absence of an indicator disease. For surveillance purposes this definition has not been accepted within the UK and Europe. In these countries AIDS continues to be a clinical diagnosis defined by one or more of the indicator diseases. The causative agent of AIDS is the human immunodeficiency virus (HIV).

Diseases diagnostic of AIDS if laboratory evidence of HIV exists

Recurrent/multiple bacterial infections—child aged under 13 years
Candidiasis—pulmonary
*Candidiasis—oesophageal
Cervical carcinoma—invasive
Coccidioidomycosis—disseminated
Cryptococcosis—pulmonary
Cryptosporidiosis—with diarrhoea persisting >1 month
*Cytomegalovirus retinitis
Cytomegalovirus disease—not in liver, spleen or nodes
HIV encephalopathy
Herpes simplex virus (HSV) infection—mucocutaneous ulceration lasting >1 month or pulmonary, oesophageal infection
Histoplasmosis—disseminated
Isosporiasis—with diarrhoea persisting >1 month
*Kaposi's sarcoma
*Lymphoid interstitial pneumonia—child aged under 13 years
Non-Hodgkins lymphoma—Burkitt's or immunoblastic
Primary cerebral lymphoma
*Disseminated mycobacteriosis—for example, *Mycobacterium avium*
*Mycobacterial tuberculosis—extrapulmonary, pulmonary
**Pneumocystis carinii* pneumonia
*Recurrent pneumonia within a 12-month period
Progressive multifocal leucoencephalopathy
Salmonella septicaemia—recurrent
*Cerebral toxoplasmosis
Wasting syndrome due to HIV

* These indicator diseases may be diagnosed presumptively

Centre for Disease Control (CDC) revised classification system for HIV infection: 1993

CD4+ T-cell categories	Clinical categories		
	(A) Asymptomatic, acute (primary) HIV or PGL	(B) Symptomatic, not (A) or (C) conditions	(C) AIDS-indicator conditions
(1) $\geqslant 500 \times 10^6/l$	A1	B1	C1
(2) $200-499 \times 10^6/l$	A2	B2	C2
(3) $< 200 \times 10^6/l$	A3	B3	C3

Diseases diagnostic of AIDS without laboratory evidence of HIV

Candidiasis—oesophageal, pulmonary
Cryptococcosis—extrapulmonary
Cytomegalovirus disease—disseminated
Cryptosporidiosis—diarrhoea persisting >1 month
Herpes simplex virus (HSV) infection —mucocutaneous ulceration lasting >1 month —pulmonary, oesophageal infection
Kaposi's sarcoma—patient aged <60 years
Primary cerebral lymphoma—patient aged <60 years
Lymphoid interstitial pneumonia—child aged <13 years
Mycobacterium avium } Disseminated
Mycobacterium kansasii
Pneumocystis carinii pneumonia
Progressive multifocal leucoencephalopathy
Cerebral toxoplasmosis

Epidemiology

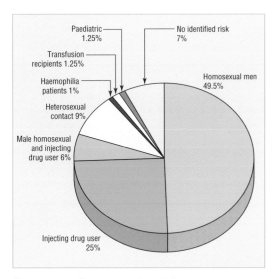

Percentage of persons with AIDS by exposure categories: USA

HIV is transmitted sexually, in blood or blood products, and perinatally. The number of reported cases continues to increase. By June 1997, 612 078 cases had been reported in the USA and by December 1997, 15 074 in the UK. Within the developed world most of those affected are men (89% in UK, 54% in USA) of whom the majority are either homosexual or injecting drug users. Most of the affected women are either injecting drug users, have had sexual contact with injecting drug users or bisexual men, or are from countries where heterosexual transmission is a prominent risk factor. Paediatric cases usually occur as a result of the mother having AIDS or belonging to a group at risk of AIDS, usually an injecting drug user. The "no identified risk" group includes people for whom information is incomplete, for example, because of death or inadequate history.

Among patients newly diagnosed HIV antibody positive every year the proportion who are heterosexual has increased. In 1997 in the USA, heterosexuals accounted for more than 50% of new diagnoses which largely reflects the epidemic amongst intravenous drug users. In contrast in the UK the increase in heterosexuals reflects acquired HIV infection in Africa. Worldwide heterosexual intercourse is the main route of transmission. In sub-Saharan Africa, South and South East Asia the ratio of infected men to infected woman is virtually 1 : 1.

In 1997 both the incidence of new cases of AIDS and the mortality rate from AIDS decreased for the first time in North America and Europe as the result of the use of more potent antiretroviral combination therapies.

Immunology

Range of immune dysfunction

- ↓ T helper cell responses
- Depletion of T-cell antigen repertoire
- ↓ Cytotoxic responses: cell-mediated T cell (CD8) natural killer cells
- ↓ Skin allergy to common recall antigens such as candida, PPD, tetanus
- ↓ Lymphocyte proliferative responses (mitogens, antigens, alloantigens)
- ↓ Monocyte function
- ↓ Immunoglobulins: polyclonal B-cell activation ↓ de novo antibody response

A depletion or impaired function of the T helper lymphocyte subset (lymphocytes bearing the CD4 cluster differentiation antigen) is the primary abnormality of immune dysfunction. The CD4 molecule, however, is also displayed at lower density on other cells such as monocytes, macrophages, and some B lymphocytes. The CD4 lymphocyte has a pivotal role in the immune response (interacting with macrophages, other T cells, B cells, and natural killer cells either by direct contact or via the influence of lymphokines such as gamma interferon and interleukin 2). The other immunological abnormalities seem to be largely secondary to the disorder of CD4 lymphocytes.

The virus

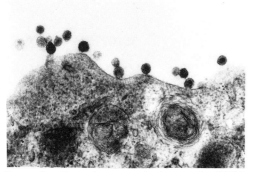

Properties: Retrovirus, two single strands of RNA, 100–120 nm diameter; genes are *gag* (core proteins), *pol* (polymerase/reverse transcriptase), *env* (envelope proteins) and accessory genes that regulate viral protein synthesis and replication; wide genomic diversity, most pronounced in *env* region. CD4 tropism; cytopathic effect in susceptible cell lines; latency; antibodies to core and envelope proteins (weak neutralising activity).

HIV has a cylindrical core. Its nucleic acid has been cloned and sequenced. It has a basic gene structure common to retroviruses but is very different from the other human retroviruses, human T lymphotropic viruses I and II. The CD4 antigen is a major component of the viral receptor required for cell entry. Only cells bearing this antigen are susceptible to infection. The beta chemokine receptors (CCR5, CXCR4) also act as coreceptors for HIV entry and their expression on the cell surface determines the susceptibility of CD4 bearing cell lines to different HIV strains. On entry to the infected cell the viral reverse transcriptase enzyme (hence retrovirus) makes a DNA copy of the RNA genome (proviral DNA). The proviral DNA is able to integrate into the host cell DNA. Latent or non-productive or productive viral replication may occur. During productive replication RNA transcripts are made from the proviral DNA, and complete virus particles are assembled and released from infected cells by characteristic budding.

In vitro, HIV produces a cytopathic effect in susceptible cell lines, multinucleate giant cells (syncytia) form, and cell death occurs.

Serological profile

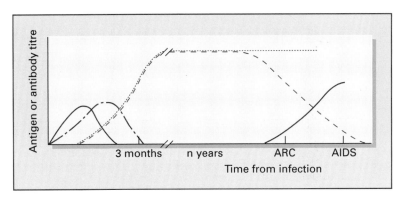

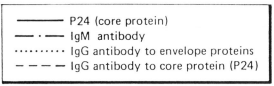

Serological profile of infection with HIV

Acute viraemia, detected by the presence of HIV RNA in plasma, precedes the appearance of antibodies (IgG and IgM) to the virus. While the patient remains asymptomatic, high titres of antibodies to envelope and core proteins persist. As immune deficiency develops the titre of antibody to the core protein (P24) falls but the titres of antibodies to the viral envelope proteins (GP 41, 120, and 160) remain high.

Molecular techniques have been developed to measure levels of plasma viral RNA and cellular viral DNA. During acute primary infection high levels of plasma viraemia are detected but decline following seroconversion. Viral RNA continues to remain detectable in plasma during the asymptomatic phase of infection and the level is predictive of the risk of progression to symptomatic disease. A high plasma RNA level is associated with a more rapid decline in CD4 count and quicker progression to symptomatic disease, while a very low level is predictive of slow or non-progression. The efficacy of the immune response during acute primary infection seems to determine the 'set point' at which viral replication is controlled over time.

Natural history

Clinical and laboratory markers associated with increased risk of progression to AIDS

Clinical
Constitutional symptoms
Oral candidiasis
Oral hairy leucoplakia

Laboratory
Simple:
  anaemia
  lymphopenia
  neutropenia
  ↑ erythrocyte sedimentation rate

Immunological:
  ↓ CD4+ lymphocyte (absolute number and percentage)
  ↓ CD4/CD8 ratio
  ↑ β_2 microglobulin

Virological:
  ↑ plasma HIV RNA

Acute infection with HIV may be accompanied by a transient non-specific illness similar to glandular fever; it includes fever, malaise, myalgia, lymphadenopathy, pharyngitis, and a rash. A transient aseptic meningoencephalitis may also occur. Most acute infections, however, are subclinical. The acute infection is accompanied by the development of antibodies to the core and surface proteins, usually in 2–6 weeks, although delayed seroconversions have been observed. Antibodies are usually detected by enzyme linked immunoassays, and their presence can be confirmed by immunofluorescence or western blot.

A chronic infection ensues. This is symptomatic in the early stages. Physical examination may show no abnormality, but about one-third of patients have persistent generalised lymphadenopathy (nodes of 1 cm or more in diameter in two or more non-contiguous extrainguinal sites, which cannot be explained by any other infection or condition). The commonest sites of lymphadenopathy are the cervical and axillary lymph nodes; it is unusual in the hilar lymph nodes. Biopsy usually shows a benign profuse follicular hyperplasia.

Later in infection non-specific constitutional symptoms develop, which may be intermittent or persistent; they include fevers, night sweats, diarrhoea, and weight loss. Patients may also be affected by several "minor" opportunistic infections or conditions that tend to affect the mucous membranes and skin, such as oral candidiasis, oral hairy leucoplakia, herpes zoster, recurrent oral or anogenital herpes simplex, and other skin conditions such as seborrhoeic dermatitis, folliculitis, impetigo, and tinea infections. This collection of symptoms and signs, which are often a prodrome to the development of major opportunistic infection or tumour, is referred to as symptomatic non AIDS or previously AIDS related complex (ARC).

Prospective cohort studies have shown that several clinical and laboratory abnormalities carry a significant predictive value for the later development of AIDS. Without therapy, about 75% of HIV infected people can be expected to develop symptomatic (CDC group B or C) disease in 9–10 years.

Tumours

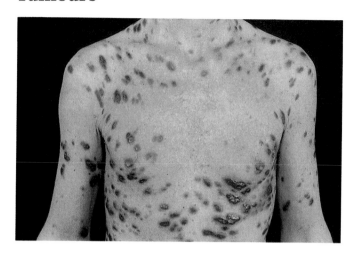

Kaposi's sarcoma

Kaposi's sarcoma (KS) is a presenting feature in 16% of patients, although the incidence has fallen over recent years. It is commoner in homosexual men than in the other groups at risk. Prior to the era of potent combination therapy, the median survival time was about 2 years, although death is usually caused by a supervening life threatening opportunistic infection.

The KS of AIDS differs from classic KS in that widespread skin, mucous membrane (particularly the oral cavity and palate), visceral, and lymph node disease occurs. Visceral, particularly gastrointestinal, lesions are present in as many as half of all patients at presentation.

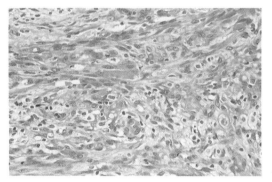

Spindle cell proliferation of nodular Kaposi's sarcoma

Nodules of KS also occur in the lungs. Chest X-ray appearances vary from confluent irregular masses to interstitial nodularity. Computed tomography of the thorax may be useful in differential diagnosis. At bronchoscopy, endobronchial lesions may be seen. KS consists of spindle shaped cells arranged in nodules and broad bands, and contains vascular slits filled with extravasated erythrocytes. The diagnosis of KS in very early skin lesions may be extremely difficult, as little more may be seen than a few irregular dilated vascular channels in the mid dermis and a mild inflammatory cell infiltrate.

More recently a new virus (human herpes virus 8, HHV8) has been identified in nearly all lesions of KS and when detected in blood predicts the later development of KS. Patient populations that have the highest risk for developing KS (homosexual/bisexual men and africans) have a high prevalence of antibodies to HHV8 and this correlates with the number of sexual partners and some past sexually transmitted infections in homosexual men. Although epidemiological evidence is supportive of sexual transmission and a causal role for HHV8 in the pathogenesis of KS, the mechanism for this has not yet been fully defined.

Non-Hodgkin's lymphoma

Extranodal disease is common and affects the central nervous system, bone marrow, and gastrointestinal tract. The diagnosis should also be considered in patients with weight loss, constitutional symptoms, and anaemia. The tumours originate from B cells, are of high or intermediate grade, and generally respond poorly to cytotoxic drugs. Squamous carcinomas of the mouth and anorectum have been described in homosexual men with antibodies to HIV. Human papillomavirus may play a part.

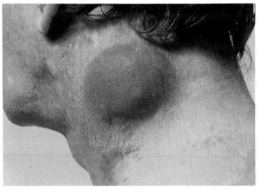

Extranodal lymphoma in the neck

Opportunistic infections

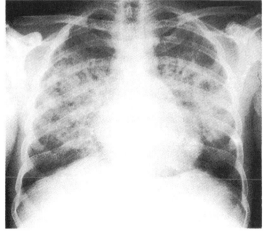

Chest radiograph of patient with typical appearances of *Pneumocystis carinii* pneumonia

The organisms responsible for the opportunistic infections occurring in patients with AIDS are unusual pathogens. Most of the infections are due to reactivation of latent organisms in the host or, in some cases, ubiquitous organisms to which we are continually exposed. The infections are often difficult to diagnose because conventional serological tests are unhelpful. Treatment often suppresses rather than eradicates the organisms. Relapses are therefore common, and continuous treatment with drugs, which may cause side effects, may be necessary.

Three main organ systems are affected: the respiratory system, the gastrointestinal tract, and the central nervous system. In addition, patients may present with a history of night sweats, chronic ill health, fevers, or weight loss.

Effect on respiratory system—typical results from bronchoscopy series

Condition	Percentage
Pneumocystis carinii pneumonia	70
Cytomegalovirus	15
Kaposi's sarcoma	5
Bacterial infection (pneumococcal, caused by *Haemophilus influenzae*, or mycobacterial (atypical or caused by *M tuberculosis*)	
Miscellaneous	5

Gastrointestinal complication of AIDS

Complications	Causes
Retrosternal discomfort and dysphagia	Candidiasis Cytomegalovirus (CMV) Herpes simplex virus (HSV)
Diarrhoea, weight loss, and malabsorption	Unknown—enteropathy Cryptosporidiosis, *Isospora belli*, and microsporidial infection CMV/HSV Mycobacteria Enteric bacteria—salmonella, campylobacter Neoplasia
Hepatitis and cholestasis	Mycobacteria CMV Drug induced Cryptosporidium
Perianal ulceration	HSV ? CMV
Neoplasia and miscellaneous	Kaposi's sarcoma Lymphoma Hairy leucoplakia Recalcitrant anorectal warts ? Squamous oral/anal carcinoma

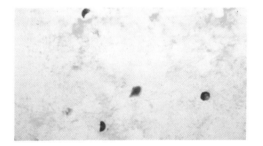

Cysts of cryptosporidium (modified Ziehl-Neelsen stain)

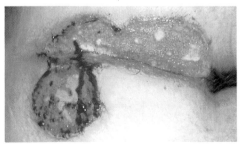

Severe mucocutaneous herpes simplex virus infection

Pulmonary complications

Pneumocystis carinii pneumonia is one of the commonest life threatening opportunistic infections in patients who progress from chronic HIV infection to AIDS. The presentation is subacute and malaise, fatigue, weight loss, and shortness of breath often develop during several weeks. Typical retrosternal or subcostal chest discomfort associated with increasing shortness of breath, a dry cough, and fever finally cause the patient to seek help. The chest radiograph at presentation may be normal or show bilateral fine infiltrates, which are typically perihilar. The arterial oxygen tension is usually depressed, and the carbon monoxide transfer factor, when available, is low and may be the earliest detectable abnormality. The diagnosis is confirmed by cytological examination of induced sputum or by fibreoptic bronchoscopy and bronchial lavage. Transbronchial biopsy is now rarely performed. Bronchoscopy can exclude other causes of pneumonia or coexistent infection such as cytomegalovirus, mycobacteria, and fungi.

Pyogenic bacterial causes of pneumonia should always be considered, particularly as its presentation may be atypical. The radiological appearances may include diffuse infiltrates as well as the more typical focal or lobar patterns. Another cause of diffuse abnormality is lymphocytic interstitial pneumonitis, more common in children than adults with AIDS.

Infection with *Mycobacterium tuberculosis* may also occur and since 1993 constitutes a diagnosis of AIDS. Among Africans presenting with AIDS it is the most common opportunistic infection and may present as pulmonary or extrapulmonary disease. In patients with advanced immunodeficiency the presentation of pulmonary tuberculosis may be atypical and should be considered in all patients with respiratory symptoms. Multi drug resistant tuberculosis occurs. Atypical mycobacteria infection may occur but usually complicates severe immune depression of advanced AIDS.

Gastrointestinal and hepatic complications

Retrosternal discomfort and dysphagia. Oral and oesophageal candidiasis is the commonest cause of dysphagia or retrosternal discomfort. Oral candidiasis alone does not fulfil the criteria for AIDS. Oesophageal infection is best shown by culture or biopsy at endoscopy, although plaques of *Candida albicans* can often be seen during a barium swallow. Ulceration may be focal or diffuse. Cytomegalovirus and herpes simplex virus may both cause a similar pattern of ulceration in the oesophagus (and also may affect the stomach and duodenum). It may be difficult to differentiate between them by barium studies.

Diarrhoea, malabsorption, and weight loss. Diarrhoea is a common symptom of patients with chronic HIV infection, with or without other manifestations of AIDS. In the majority of cases a pathogen is found though an enteropathy with malabsorption has been described secondary to HIV infection.

Cryptosporidium is a coccidian protozoal parasite and probably the commonest pathogen isolated from patients with AIDS who have diarrhoea. It is the commonest of the protozoal causes of diarrhoea, which also include *Isospora belli* and microsporidia. In immunocompetent human hosts cryptosporidium produces a transient diarrhoeal illness. In people infected with HIV it can cause transient, intermittent, or persistent diarrhoea, ranging from loose stools to watery diarrhoea, colic, and severe fluid and electrolyte loss. Oocysts can be found in stools. If direct smears of unconcentrated faecal samples stained with iodine or modified acid fast stains fail to show the oocysts the samples should be concentrated. The diagnosis should not be discounted without examining multiple specimens.

With improved diagnostic techniques microsporidia, small obligate intracellular protozoa, have been increasingly identified as a common cause of diarrhoea in patients with AIDS where no other pathogen had previously been found.

Cytomegalovirus and herpes simplex virus can cause focal or diffuse ulceration of the gut, from the mouth to the anus. Herpes simplex virus most commonly causes mucocutaneous lesions at the upper and the lower ends of the gastrointestinal tract, whereas cytomegalovirus may mimic inflammatory bowel disease.

Atypical mycobacteria of the avium intracellular complex are ubiquitous organisms that have little virulence for the immunocompetent host. Disseminated infection of several organs occurs in patients with AIDS. Gastrointestinal infection may be associated with fever, weight loss, diarrhoea, and malabsorption. Diagnosis can be made by acid fast staining of the stool or biopsy material, or both, or culture of blood or tissue. *Mycobacterium tuberculosis* infection of the bowel does occur, but is less common. *Campylobacter* and *Salmonella* species infections may cause diarrhoea, but the latter more commonly presents as a fever of unknown origin with bacteraemia.

Hepatitis and cholestasis. Hepatitis in patients with AIDS may present as fever, abdominal pain, and hepatomegaly, and liver function test results, particularly raised alkaline phosphatase activity, may be abnormal. If ultrasound does not show dilated bile ducts, needle biopsy often shows granulomatous hepatitis, usually caused by atypical mycobacteria rather than *M tuberculosis*. The herpes viruses may also occasionally cause hepatitis as part of a disseminated infection. When multiple drugs are being taken, drug induced hepatitis must always be considered, as should coinfection with hepatitis B or C particularly among homosexual/bisexual men or injecting drug users.

Acalculous cholecystis and cholangitis show an endoscopic retrograde cholangiographic picture similar to that of primary sclerosing cholangitis, with strictures and dilatation of the biliary tree. Cryptosporidium and cytomegalovirus have been shown or isolated and are implicated as a cause of this syndrome.

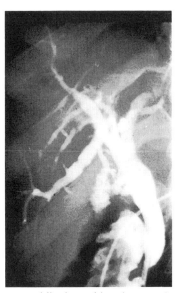

Dilated common bile duct with stricture at lower end and irregularities of extrahepatic and intrahepatic ducts

Neurological complications

Chronic HIV infection is associated with several syndromes affecting the nervous system, in addition to the transient meningoencephalitis, myelopathy, and peripheral neuropathy of acute infection. These neurological diseases are believed to be due to the direct or indirect effects of HIV and not to opportunistic infection. AIDS related dementia, now referred to as "HIV associated motor cognitive complex", has been estimated to occur in 10–40% of patients with symptomatic disease. At necropsy up to 90% of patients dying of AIDS have chronic subcortical encephalitis characterised by infected macrophages and microglial cells that fuse to form multinucleate giant cells. There is also patchy demyelination and astrogliosis.

The clinical features are characterised by cognitive and behaviourial changes that include memory loss, apathy, and impaired concentration and attention. Neurological examination may show hyperreflexia, hypertonia, and frontal release signs. Computed tomography or magnetic resonance imaging often show cerebral atrophy and non-specific changes in the white matter. The cerebrospinal fluid findings are non-specific. Opportunistic infections, intracranial mass lesions, metabolic encephalopathy, and neurosyphilis should be excluded.

HIV infection is also implicated in vacuolar myelopathy affecting primarily the posterior and lateral spinal cord, meningitis, and the following neuropathies: axonal sensory, chronic inflammatory demyelinating, and mononeuropathies. Cytomegalovirus infection may produce a polyradiculopathy.

The nervous system is also affected by opportunistic infection and tumour. Cerebral toxoplasmosis is the commonest cause of intracranial mass lesions and usually presents with focal symptoms and signs. Cytomegalovirus commonly causes a retinitis and presents with blurring or partial loss of vision, or both. It may eventually lead to blindness.

Rough incidence of conditions in patients with neurological complications

Central nervous system (CNS)	Percentage
Viral infections	
AIDS-related dementia	16
HIV-related meningitis	13
CMV retinitis	5
CMV encephalitis	2
Progressive multifocal leucoencephalopathy	0·5
Vacuolar myelopathy	4*
Intracranial mass lesions	
Cerebral toxoplasmosis	14
Primary CNS lymphoma	4
Undefined mass lesions	3
Lymphoma	1
Peripheral nervous system	
Sensory neuropathy	16
Inflammatory demyelinating neuropathy	6
Cranial neuropathies	2
Multiple mononeuropathies	1
Polyradiculopathy	2
Miscellaneous	
Cryptococcal meningitis	6
Neurosyphilis	0·5
Metabolic encephalopathy	3
Cerebrovascular accident	0·5

* May be as high as 20% at necropsy.

Protozoal opportunistic infections

Infection	Drug	Duration	Side effects	Comments
Pneumocystis carinii pneumonia Treatment	Co-trimoxazole (trimethoprim component 20 mg/kg/day) intravenously for 14 days then orally	14–21 days	Nausea, fever, rash, bone marrow suppression	80% of patients will respond to treatment
	OR pentamidine isethionate 4 mg/kg/day or pentamidine mesylate 2.5 mg/kg/day, both as slow intravenous infusion	14–21 days	Hypotension, hypoglycaemia, renal failure, hepatitis, bone marrow suppression	
	OR clindamycin 600 mg 4 times a day	14–21 days	Nausea, diarrhoea, rash, hepatitis	For treatment of mild or moderate PCP only
	AND primaquine 30 mg once daily		Nausea, methaemoglobinaemia, haemolytic anaemia, leucopenia	
Maintenance	Co-trimoxazole 960 mg a day or on alternate days	Indefinite	Usually minimal	In the presence of positive toxoplasma serology co-trimoxazole or dapsone in combination with pyrimethamine is recommended
	OR dapsone 50–100 mg once daily or 100 mg 3 times per week			
	OR nebulised pentamidine isethionate 8 mg/kg every 2–4 weeks			
Toxoplasmosis	Pyrimethamine 50 mg/day orally and either sulphadiazine 4–6 g/day orally or clindamycin 600 mg four times/day	Indefinite	Rash, nausea, bone marrow suppression	Doses usually halved during maintenance
Cryptosporidiosis	Paromomycin 500 mg 4 times a day	28 days	Epigastric pain, dysphagia	Although observational studies report clinical improvement paromomycin is an unlicensed medication
Microsporidiosis	Albendazole 400 mg twice daily	28 days	Raised liver function tests, headache, gastrointestinal disturbance	Observational studies report improved clinical outcome but treatment of microsporidiosis is an unlicensed indication for albendazole

Viral opportunistic infections

Infection	Drug	Duration	Side effects	Comments
Herpes simplex Treatment	Acyclovir 200 mg 5 times a day orally or 5–10 mg/kg 8 hourly intravenously	10–14 days		
Prophylaxis	Acyclovir 200 mg four times a day	Indefinite		May be possible to reduce frequency
Cytomegalovirus Treatment	Ganciclovir 5 mg/kg twice a day	14–21 days	Anaemia, neutropenia	Marrow suppression potentiated with zidovudine
	OR foscarnet 90 mg/kg twice a day	14–21 days	Nephrotoxicity, hypocalcaemia, headache	Dose titrated to creatinine clearance
	OR cidofovir 5 mg/kg/weekly	2 weeks	Nephrotoxicity, hypocalcaemia	Pre and post dosing with probenecid limits risk of nephrotoxicity
Maintenance	Ganciclovir 2.5–5 mg/kg/day	Indefinite	Anaemia, neutropenia	
	OR foscarnet 90 mg /kg/day	Indefinite	See above	See above
	OR cidofovir 5 mg/kg/per 2 weeks	Indefinitely	See above	See above

Fungal opportunistic infections

Infection	Drug	Duration	Side effects	Comments
Candidiasis Local treatment	Nystatin oral suspension or pastilles, miconazole oral gel, or amphotericin lozenges all 4–6 times a day	As required		Relapse common, many patients require systemic treatment
Systemic treatment	Ketoconazole 200–400 mg a day orally	7–14 days	Nausea, hepatitis, thrombocytopenia	Relapse common on cessation of treatment
	OR Fluconazole 50–200 mg/day	7–14 days	Hepatitis	Relapse common on cessation of treatment
	OR Itraconazole 200–400 mg/day	7–14 days	Hepatitis	Relapse common on cessation of treatment
Maintenance	Fluconazole 50–100 mg/day or alternate days	Indefinite	Nausea, hepatitis	Clinical resistance may occur in patients with advanced disease
	OR Itraconazole 200 mg/day			
Cryptococcosis Treatment	Amphotericin B 0.3 mg/kg/day and flucytosine 150 mg/kg/day in 4 doses	6 weeks	Nausea, vomiting, rash, bone marrow suppression, renal damage, hypocalcaemia	Liposomal preparations of amphotericin associated with reduced risk of nephrotoxicity
	OR fluconazole 400–800 mg/day	6 weeks	Nausea, hepatitis	
Maintenance	Fluconazole 200–400 mg/day	Indefinite	See above	
	OR amphotericin 1 mg/kg twice weekly	Indefinite	See above	

Treatment

Dideoxynucleosides

T

5′
HOCH2 O
4   1   Thymidine
3′ 2
OH

T

5′
HOCH2 O
4   1   3′–Azido–3′–deoxythmidin
3′ 2

N3

C

5′
HOCH2 O
4   1   2′–deoxycytidine
3′ 2
OH

C

5′
HOCH2 O
4   1   2′–3′ dideoxycytidine
3′ 2

H

Reverse transcriptase inhibitors

Nucleoside analogues:	Non-nucleoside analogues:
Zidovudine	Nevirapine
Stavudine	Delavadine
Didanosine	Efavirenz
Zalcitabine	
Lamivudine	
Abacavir	

Protease inhibitors

Indinavir
Nelfinavir
Saquinavir
Ritonavir
Amprenavir

Antiretrovirals

Therapy for HIV infection has greatly improved in the last 2–3 years with the development of potent combination regimens that effectively reduce plasma HIV RNA levels and increase CD4 counts, resulting in substantial clinical benefit in terms of a decreased mortality and morbidity. In 1997 the incidence in developed countries of new AIDS defining illnesses and the AIDS related mortality rate fell between 30% and 50% as a result of the widespread use of combination therapies.

Three main classes of antiretroviral drugs are available for inclusion in treatment regimens. The nucleoside analogues and a variety of non-nucleoside agents inhibit the viral reverse transcriptase enzyme which produces a DNA copy from the single strand of viral RNA. The protease inhibitors inhibit post-translational processing of viral proteins. Combinations of two nucleoside reverse transcriptase inhibitors (RTIs) and one protease inhibitor have been shown in clinical trials to decrease progression to AIDS and improve survival in patients with relatively advanced disease to a greater extent than a combination of two nucleoside RTIs alone.

In terms of AIDS progression and survival the clinical effectiveness of the non-nucleoside RTIs in combination regimens has not yet been demonstrated but combinations of two nucleosides and one non-nucleoside RTIs have been shown to result in similar falls in plasma viral RNA and increases in CD4 count over 1 year of treatment to that seen with some protease inhibitor containing regimens. Combinations of non-nucleoside RTIs and protease inhibitors are being evaluated in clinical trials.

The data from large randomised clinical studies have shown an association between falls in plasma HIV RNA levels in the short term and clinical benefit after 1–2 years of follow up. The greater the level of viral suppression the greater the reduction in risk of clinical progression. Monitoring of both CD4 counts and plasma HIV RNA levels is essential for assessing the effectiveness of a given combination regimen. Optimal responses may be measured in terms of reduction and maintenance of plasma HIV RNA levels to below the level of detectability of the assay; however, this may not always be achieved and a substantial reduction in plasma HIV RNA levels is associated with clinical benefit. Despite effective combination treatments, rebound in plasma HIV RNA levels occurs frequently. Factors which might contribute to this include the emergence of drug resistance virus, non-adherence to combination treatment regimens, malabsorption of drugs, and pharmacological failure. For the non-nucleoside RTIs and the currently licensed protease inhibitors viral resistance to one drug is associated with cross resistance to others in the same class, limiting the effectiveness of different combinations and reducing future therapeutic options. Avoidance of drug resistance is likely to be important in sustaining an antiviral effect. Assays to detect both phenotype and genotype have been developed and their use in routine clinical practice is being evaluated.

Early data suggests that effective control of viral replication results in immunological improvements in terms of the number and phenotype of T cells, lymphocyte proliferative responses and lymph node architecture, but the long-term duration of clinical benefit from combination regimens is uncertain.

On current data the optimum time to start a therapy is unknown, but factors which influence the decision to start include the risk of clinical progression as determined by the CD4 count, plasma HIV RNA level and presence or not of symptoms, the efficacy, tolerability and long-term toxicity of drug regimens and not least the willingness and ability of the patient to start and comply with treatment regimens.

Opportunistic infections and tumours

Conventional cytotoxic drugs and radiotherapy are used for Kaposi' sarcoma. Alfa interferon has also been used. All induce remission in some cases but none alter median survival. Some regimens carry increased risks of opportunistic infection and side effects that affect the quality of life considerably.

Advances in managing and preventing opportunistic infections have also occurred and contributed significantly to the improvement and survival of patients with symptomatic disease that has occurred since 1987. The use of primary prophylaxis against *Pneumocystis carinii* pneumonia has resulted in its decreased incidence as an AIDS defining diagnosis. Similar primary prophylactic strategies have also influenced the development of cerebral toxoplasmosis and disseminated Mycobacterium Avium Intracellulare infection. Although antimicrobial prophylaxis is an essential part of treatment strategy, the use of potent combination therapies, particularly protease inhibitors in patients with advanced disease, has had a major impact on the incidence of opportunistic infections and their natural history.

It has been possible for some patients who have had significant improvements in immunological function on combination regimens to stop secondary prophylaxis for opportunistic infections. Widespread use of this strategy when it is clear that immunological recovery is slow in response to current combination regimens would be unwise until there is more data.

Prevention and control

Prevention and control

- Surveillance
- Counselling and health education
- (a) Screening of people and donated blood
  (b) Heat treatment of blood products
- Protection of health-care staff

As no cure or vaccine is currently available, our main weapon is prevention and control. An "information vaccine" is required. In any epidemic an accurate appreciation of the size of the problem and how it is changing is essential. With HIV infection this can be achieved by counting the number of patients with AIDS and monitoring the prevalence of antibody of HIV in low- and high-risk populations.

Of fundamental importance is good and accurate health education for those at low risk and those at high risk. People who may have been exposed are advised not to donate blood, organs, or semen, and to modify their sexual behaviour to avoid practices that are particularly likely to transmit the virus. The screening of blood donors for antibody to HIV and the heat treatment of blood products have virtually eliminated the risk to recipients.

GENITAL WARTS AND MOLLUSCUM CONTAGIOSUM

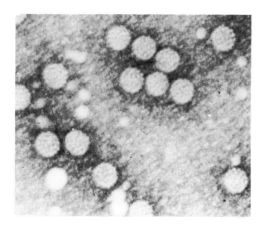

Even though genital warts (condyloma acuminatum) are commonly seen in departments of genitourinary medicine (about 97 000 cases a year) many more cases are diagnosed and treated by general practitioners, surgeons, gynaecologists, and dermatologists. Not only are warts common but they are difficult and time consuming to treat.

They are caused by a small DNA virus, a papillomavirus belonging to the papovavirus group, which cannot be cultured. Genital warts differ from skin warts histologically and antigenically and are most commonly caused by types 6 or 11. Types 16, 18, 31, 33, and 35 also cause genital warts. Genital warts are nearly always transmitted by sexual contact; autoinoculation from hand to genitals is unusual. Infants and young children may develop laryngeal papillomas due to infection from maternal genital warts at delivery. The infectivity of sexually acquired warts is about 60%; the incubation period is long, varying from two weeks to eight months (mean three months).

Clinical features

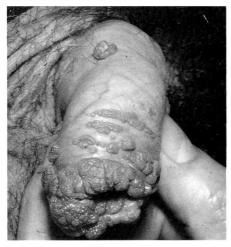

Genital warts are often asymptomatic and painless. Patients may give a history of suddenly noticing them or noticing them only once their sexual contact has acquired them. Women are more likely to be unaware of warts because it is harder for them to examine their genitalia. Warts flourish in warm, moist conditions, particularly if a discharge or other infections are present.

Warts may be solitary but are usually multiple by the time the patient attends for consultation. In men they may be found on the glans and shaft of the penis, prepuce, fraenum and coronal sulcus, urethral meatus, scrotum, anus, and rectum. In women the commonest site of infection is the introitus and vulva, but warts may also affect the vagina and (as flat warts) the cervix. Other infected sites may be the perineum, anus, and rectum.

Warts—penile, intrameatal, vulval, and perianal

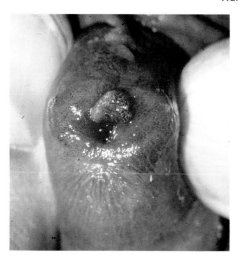 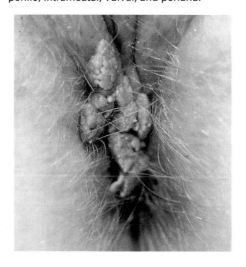 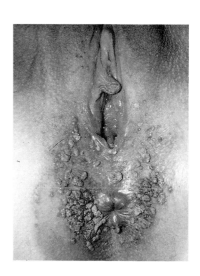

Diagnosis

Genital warts are one of the few sexually transmitted conditions that are diagnosed solely from their clinical features. Diagnosis is not usually difficult but the differential diagnosis of condylomata lata of secondary syphilis, molluscum contagiosum, sebaceous cysts, and benign and malignant tumours should be remembered. Warts may often herald other sexually transmitted diseases or infections. For example, one third of women attending departments of genitourinary medicine with genital warts have one or more additional diseases diagnosed concurrently. All women with genital warts, even in the absence of any other symptoms, must have a full set of microbiological tests performed to exclude infection with *Candida albicans*, *Trichomonas vaginalis*, *Neisseria gonorrhoeae*, *Chlamydia trachomatis*, and bacterial vaginosis. Heterosexual and homosexual men with penile warts should have urethral tests for gonorrhoea, *C trachomatis* and non-gonococcal urethritis, even if they are asymptomatic. Likewise, homosexuals with anal warts should have proctoscopy performed to exclude the presence of additional warts within the rectum as well as other rectal diseases such as gonorrhoea. Finally, serological tests for syphilis should be carried out in both men and women. Contact tracing and examination of regular sexual partners must be undertaken as well as full microbiological investigations for other STDs.

Differential diagnosis of genital warts
● Condylomata lata
● Molluscum contagiosum
● Sebaceous cysts
● Tumours

Complications

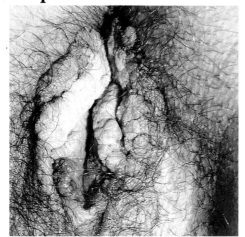

Massive warts in pregnancy

Complications of genital warts are rare. Occasionally they may increase alarmingly in size during pregnancy and appear as large cauliflower-like masses. In men similar giant benign but destructive warts (Buschke-Lowenstein tumour) may occur on the penis or existing small ones may rapidly become enlarged. Malignant transformation of vulval, cervical, penile, and anal warts has been reported.

Flat warts on the cervix are not usually apparent to the naked eye. Cervical dysplasia is strongly associated with HPV types 16, 18, 31, 33, and 35 and in particular types 16 and 18. Therefore all women who have had genital warts should have regular cytology performed once a year.

Treatment

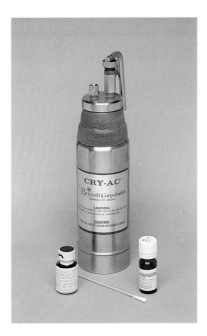

Initial treatment is usually with locally applied caustic agents. It is usual to start with podophyllin—a cytotoxic agent—which should be applied to the lesions in strengths of 10% or 25% in industrial spirit and repeated at least twice or even three times a week. Being an irritating substance it can cause bad burns. Patients must therefore be told to wash it off three to four hours after application. Patients may often want to apply podophyllin themselves, but this is undesirable, since they may be overzealous in their justifiable desire to get rid of their warts and apply the substance too often, without washing it off, on the basis that "if it hurts it must be doing me good." Severe systemic effects of peripheral neuropathy, coma, and hypokalaemia can follow application of large quantities. Podophyllotoxin 0·5% has less severe side effects and can be used by the patient for application at home. The patient is told to administer this twice a day for three days and to repeat this four days later if necessary.

If podoyphyllin applied regularly is ineffective after two to three weeks the more caustic agent glacial trichloroacetic acid 50–100% may be used, again with great caution. This agent is more often used for hyperkeratotic warts but even so these warts are often resistant and electrocautery or cryotherapy (cryoprobe or cryac spray) will be needed. Cautery or surgical excision should be considered at an earlier stage if the warts are particularly large or numerous. The clinical course of warts, particularly their ability to regress spontaneously and reappear, has made other treatment regimens— such as vaccines, fluorouracil, and interferon—difficult to assess.

Approaches to the treatment of genital warts

Site or type of warts	Start	1 week	2 weeks	3 weeks	4 weeks
Few, small, and soft	10–25% Podophyllin or podophyllotoxin	→	→	Trichloracetic acid	Cryotherapy electrocautery
Solitary, large, discrete	Electrocautery diathermy, excision, cryotherapy				
Extensive, multiple, vegetations	10–25% Podophyllin or podophyllotoxin or Trichloracetic acid	→	Surgical excision		
Hyperkeratotic	Trichloracetic acid or cryotherapy	→	Electrocautery diathermy		
Intrameatal	Cryotherapy	→	Electrocautery cryotherapy		
Cervical	Colposcopy, cryotherapy, laser				
Vaginal	Cryotherapy				
Anal	Cryotherapy				
Pregnancy	None—unless discrete small vaginal or vulval, then use trichloracetic acid/cryotherapy-? electrocautery				

During pregnancy it is best to offer no treatment. Podophyllin is contraindicated in view of its toxicity and possible mutagenic action, and the warts usually diminish in size once pregnancy has ended. Trichloracetic acid may be used if the lesions are discrete and small and occur on the vaginal wall or vulva. Alternatively, cryotherapy or electrocautery may be offered. Occasionally caesarean section is necessary if the warts are likely to obstruct labour. Laryngeal papilloma can occur in neonates, infants and children, possibly transmitted transplacentally, perinatally or postnatally. Whether these are prevented by treatment of the mother during pregnancy is not known, and is certainly not an indication on its own for caesarean section.

Doctors treating genital warts outside sexually transmitted disease clinics should remember, firstly, that an accurate and detailed sexual history is needed; secondly, that concurrent sexually acquired conditions should be excluded; and, thirdly, that contact tracing must be carried out.

Treatment of warts outside departments of genitourinary medicine

- Sexual history

- Exclude a concurrent sexually transmitted disease

- Trace regular sexual contacts

Molluscum contagiosum

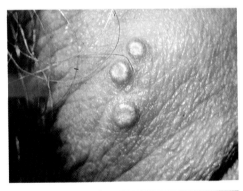

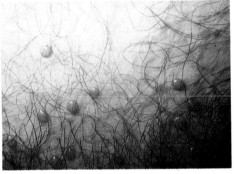

Molluscum contagiosum may be transmitted sexually but this is not the only route. It is a contagious viral condition which may be spread by close bodily contact, clothing, or towels. Transmission (outbreaks) is possible in swimming pools, sauna baths, schools, after massage, and between siblings. The agent causing molluscum contagiosum is one of the pox viruses and has a variable incubation period of two to twelve weeks. Cases are seen in clinics but far more are probably seen by general practitioners and dermatologists.

Clinical features—The lesions of molluscum contagiosum are characteristic. The pearly white umbilicated papules appear in the genital area (penis, scrotum, vulva, perineum, abdomen, and thighs), but if transmission is non-sexual they may also be found in any part of the body but particularly on the arms, face, eyelids, and scalp. The lesions are usually small (2–5 mm in diameter).

Diagnosis is usually based on the clinical appearance since the virus cannot be grown successfully. Material expressed from the centre of lesions shows viral inclusions in Giemsa stain or on electron microscopy. Since the condition may be sexually transmitted other infections similarly spread should be excluded if the patient's history or the site of the lesions (proximity to genital area) suggests that this could be the route of infection.

Treatment is by applying phenol on the end of a sharpened stick to the central umbilicated core of the lesions. This may need to be repeated several times. Alternatively electrocautery or cryotherapy may be used.

GENITAL INFESTATIONS

Pediculosis pubis

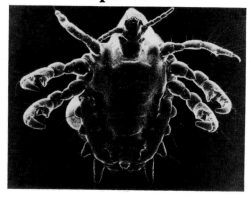

Pediculosis pubis is caused by the pubic louse, *Phthirus pubis*, which is a different species from that causing head and body louse infestation (pediculosis capitis and corporis). The insect is small and round (1–2 mm long) and has three sets of legs. The adult adheres not only to pubic hair but also to other hairy areas (perinium, thighs, abdomen, axillas, eyebrows, and eyelashes) and is a blood sucker. The female lays eggs (nits) at the base of the hairs and these usually hatch within seven days. The adult louse is transferred from person to person during close bodily contact. Since lice do not leave the host the condition is not spread by wearing or sleeping in infested clothing or sheets. The patient may complain of irritation. Sometimes the condition is asymptomatic and the patient may be horrified to find the adult louse or nits on the body.

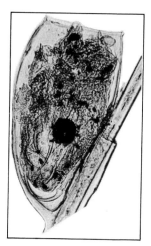

Diagnosis is usually based on clinical appearances alone. A hand lens is useful during the examination and a suspected louse on a hair may be removed and viewed under the low power microscope. Bluish grey macules occasionally occur on the abdomen, buttocks, or thighs at the site of the bites. As the condition is usually sexually acquired a full genitourinary and sexual history must be taken and the patient examined for other sexually transmitted diseases. Blood must also be taken for syphilis serology.

Treatment—0·5% Malathion (Derbac M) or 1% gamma benzene hexachloride powder (Gammexane) should be applied to all the hairy areas apart from the scalp. The patient should not wash this off for 24 hours, after which a bath should be taken. Usually one application is enough, but a heavy infestation will necessitate further treatment within 7–10 days. Alternatively 1% gamma benzene hexachloride can be used as a cream or lotion (Lorexane, Quellada) or carbaryl as 0·5% lotion (Carylderm, Clinicide, Suleo-c, Derbac Shampoo). Patient's clothes and bed linen should be washed in hot water or dry cleaned. Sexual partners should also be seen and treated. Shaving of body hair is not necessary.

Gamma benzene hexachloride should not be used in pregnant women since it is lipid soluble and can be stored in body fat and appear in breast milk.

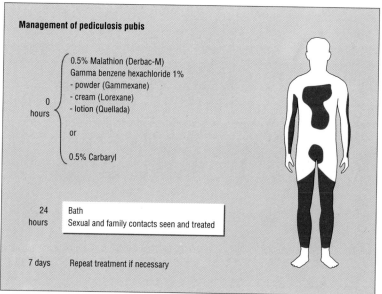

Management of pediculosis pubis

0 hours	0.5% Malathion (Derbac-M) Gamma benzene hexachloride 1% - powder (Gammexane) - cream (Lorexane) - lotion (Quellada) or 0.5% Carbaryl
24 hours	Bath Sexual and family contacts seen and treated
7 days	Repeat treatment if necessary

Scabies

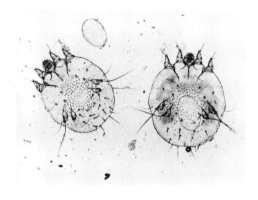

Infestation is caused by the mite *Sarcoptes scabiei*. The clinical features of scabies are caused by the female burrowing into the uppermost layer of the skin (stratum corneum) and laying eggs and defecating. The female is about twice the size (0·3 mm long) of the male and can just be seen by the naked eye as a black dot (mouth parts) at the distal part of the burrow. Infestation usually occurs as a result of close physical, but not necessarily sexual, contact. This needs to be reasonably prolonged since the insect moves slowly, at 25 mm a minute. Outbreaks of non-sexually acquired scabies may occur among schoolchildren and within whole households or long stay hospitals.

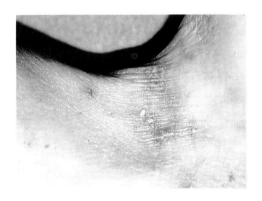

Symptoms are first noticed two to six weeks after infestation. Reinfection may give rise to symptoms within a few hours. The patient complains of itching, which is often unbearable, intractable, and worse at night when the body is warm. The sites of itching and burrows bear no relation to the mode of transmission. Thus lesions may often be found in the clefts of fingers and on the wrists and elbows as well as on the genitals. On examination the burrows may be the typical sinuous scaling reddish grey lesions (5–15 mm long), sometimes with small vesicles at their end. Scratching may, however, alter their appearance, with excoriation, ulceration, crusting, and bleeding; on the penis and scrotum they may appear as red papules. Associated rashes may also be found in sites distant from the actual burrows—in particular erythematous urticarial papules in the armpits, abdominal wall, and the anterior and posterior aspects of the upper thighs. In some cases indurated nodules, eczematous changes, and secondary infection with pustule formation may occur.

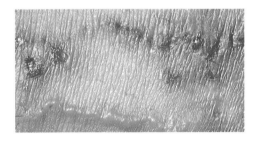

Diagnosis is based on the clinical history and examination and may be confirmed by finding the mite. This is achieved by scraping the top off the whole length of a burrow (from distal to proximal end) with a scalpel, putting the material on a slide with 10% potassium hydroxide solution, and looking for the mite under the microscope. As with pediculosis pubis, if the history suggests sexual transmission other sexually transmitted diseases must be excluded.

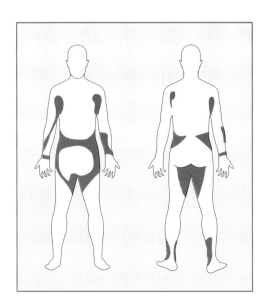

Treatment—Scabies is treated by the application of 0·5% malathion (Derbac-M) or permethrin 5% (Lyclear) which should be applied to the whole body. Patients should be told that the initial itching may persist for several weeks despite successful treatment with either preparation. Unless this explanation is given patients may equate the symptoms with continuing infection, retreat themselves, and run the risk of a chemical dermatitis. Sexual contacts should be seen if sexual transmission is suspected; if the condition was not acquired by this route other members of the family or school friends will need to be treated. When contacts are seen they may be asymptomatic but should be treated since they may be incubating the disease. No special treatment of clothing or bed linen is necessary.

Tinea cruris

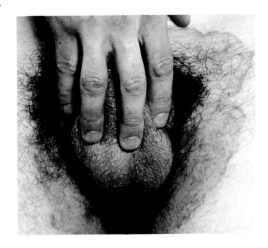

Management

Normally:	Clotrimazole, miconazole, or econazole cream
Resistant/ relasping:	Terbinafine 250 mg daily for 2–4 weeks
	Itraconazole 100 mg daily for 15 days

Tinea cruris is a common skin condition, particularly in men. If limited to the groin area it is caused by one of two fungi—*Trichophyton rubrum* or *Epidermophyton floccosum*. The patient may complain of an irritating rash, particularly in the groin. When patients attend a department of genitourinary medicine with this condition they may be extremely distraught because they fear that the condition is sexually acquired or even, having read about rashes, fear that it could be due to syphilis. The same type of patient consulting doctors outside the clinics may regard the condition as no more than a "sweat rash."

The rash has a scaly, marginated, erythematous appearance, the edges of which are occasionally vesicular or pustular. It needs to be differentiated from a seborrhoeic or contact dermatitis, psoriasis, and candidiasis. The diagnosis is based on the clinical history and appearance and may be confirmed by mixing scrapings of the lesions with 10% potassium hydroxide solution and viewing them under a normal microscope, when mycelium can be seen. The fungi may be cultured on Sabouraud's medium. Imidazole derivatives can be applied as a cream (clotrimazole, miconazole, econazole). This is applied once or twice daily until the lesions disappear and should be continued for a further one to two weeks to avoid reappearance. In severe resistant or relapsing cases terbinafine 250 mg daily for two to four weeks can be used. Also itraconazole 100 mg daily for 15 days can be prescribed. Both of these drugs may need to be continued for longer periods of time.

GENITAL SKIN AND OTHER CONDITIONS

- Lichen sclerosus et atrophicus

- Lichen planus

- Psoriasis and dermatitis

- Dermatitis

- Trauma

- Lymphocele

- Peyronie's disease

Several skin and other conditions may affect the genital area but are not sexually transmitted. Because of their anatomical site patients with these conditions seek medical advice in the fear that they have acquired a sexually transmitted disease.

Lichen sclerosus et atrophicus

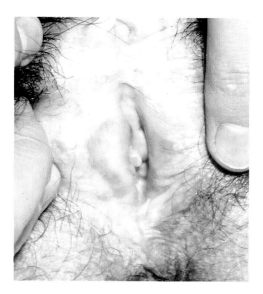

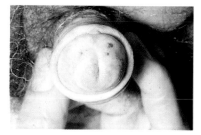

Lichen sclerosus et atrophicus is a rare disease that may occur in any age group but usually in those aged 30–60 years. The aetiology is unknown. The skin in the affected areas is atrophic, with white plaques and eventual contraction of tissues. When localised to the male genitals the condition is called balanitis xerotica obliterans. In men the major sites affected are the glans penis, urethral meatus with extension into the terminal urethra, and the prepuce. In women the changes are found on the vulva, vaginal introitus, clitoris, perineum, and anus.

Clinical features—Men with this condition may present with penile pain and irritation, urethral discharge, and in the later stages of the disease phimosis and urinary obstruction. Women may notice itching of the vulva, sometimes associated with superficial dyspareunia. The dyspareunia may also be due to lesions on the vaginal introitus. The condition should not be forgotten as one of the causes of persistent pruritus vulvae.

On examination white plaques may be seen on the glans and prepuce, often encircling the end of the foreskin, which may be difficult to retract. The urethral meatus may also be surrounded with a small collar of white tissue extending a small distance up the urethra so that the first centimetre is pipe stem hard and the meatus very small in size. In women the same type of plaques may be found on the vulva, and the skin may often appear thin, with a parchment quality, and shiny. These skin changes may affect other areas of the body. In some cases erythema, purpura, excoriations, blister formation, and pigmentary changes may also be seen.

Diagnosis and treatment—The diagnosis should be confirmed by biopsy and histology. The aim of treatment is both to relieve the symptoms and to slow down the disease process. This may often be achieved by the application of a potent topical corticosteroid cream twice a day. In addition the skin may be moisturised and softened by the use of aqueous cream *BP* as a soap substitute and moisturising cream. Long term follow up is recommended since the lesions, particularly the phimosis and meatal narrowing, may progress and require dilatation, meatotomy, or circumcision. Neoplastic changes (squamous cell carcinoma) of the lesions may occur later.

Lichen planus

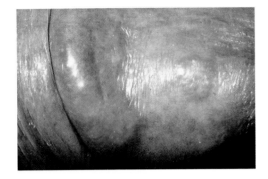

Lichen planus affects the genital area and other parts of the body and may present with mauvish papules or plaques. Usually the patient complains of itching at the site of the lesions, which occur on the glans penis, shaft, foreskin, scrotum, vulva, and perianal areas. The lesions may be papular or annular and are often white, particularly if situated in moist parts of the body. They may also be found in extragenital areas such as the arms, flexor aspects of the wrists, legs, and buccal epithelium. The disease is eventually self limiting but some relief can be obtained with a topical corticosteroid cream or ointment.

Psoriasis

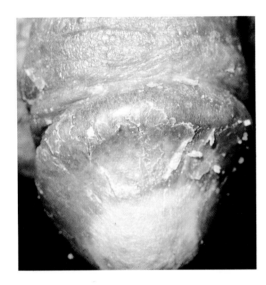

Psoriasis may affect the genital area either alone or in conjunction with widespread disease elsewhere. The lesions of psoriasis may be found on the penis, scrotum, vulva, groins, perineum, and perianal areas. These are often similar to the scaly red psoriasiform lesions found in other parts of the body. They may, however, lose their scales if present in moist parts of the genitalia and appear red and shiny. The condition has to be differentiated from tinea cruris, candidiasis, lichen planus, keratodermia blennorrhagia, erythroplasia, and seborrhoeic or contact dermatitis. In relation to the sexually transmitted diseases the most important condition that may look the same is the scaly papular rash of secondary syphilis. The presence of psoriasis in non-genital areas and the nails will help to exclude syphilis, however, though patients with psoriasis may also have syphilis. Psoriasis and dermatitis are not contagious but in patients presenting with skin conditions affecting the genital area it is essential to bear in mind that such conditions could be sexually acquired and to examine the entire surface of the skin.

The treatment of psoriasis affecting the genital region is the same as that for the condition in general.

Dermatitis

Factors causing contact dermatitis

- Soaps
- Deodorants
- Forms of clothing
- Medicaments
- Condoms
- Friction or trauma

There are two common types of dermatitis of the genitalia— seborrhoeic or contact. Seborrhoeic dermatitis is only rarely localised to the genital area, and other areas such as the scalp, ears, chest, axillas, and back may be affected. The lesions are red and scaly and not well circumscribed. Again all skin areas must be examined. The condition is not related to any known precipitating factors and in this way differs from contact dermatitis. On careful questioning patients with contact dermatitis may relate their symptoms to the use of particular soaps, deodorants, forms of clothing, medicaments, and occasionally the sheath or to friction and trauma. They may complain of irritation possibly associated with swelling. Unless the patient is examined during the acute phase there will be little to see apart from mild erythema. Should the contact dermatitis continue, however, thickening and scaling of the skin may occur. Patch testing is likely to be needed to confirm the diagnosis if there is a possibility of an allergic contact dermatitis.

The symptomatic treatment of dermatitis is usually with topical corticosteroid preparations. In contact dermatitis the causative agent should be removed.

Trauma

- Deliberate   Atypical lesions

                     Bizarre appearance

                     Accessible to patient's hand

                     Psychiatric assessment

- Accidental   Atypical lesions

                     Mechanical instruments

                     Surgical repair
                     (occasionally)

Several genital conditions, such as trauma, lymphocele, and Peyronie's disease, may be alarming both to the doctor and the patient. Trauma to the genitalia may be purposely or accidentally inflicted. Purposely self inflicted trauma (dermatitis artefacta) should be suspected when atypical lesions are present. They look bizarre, do not resemble any known condition, and are found in areas accessible to the patient's hand. The patient, who usually denies the aetiology, is often mentally unstable, and psychiatric assessment and help are needed.

The number of cases of accidental self inflicted genital trauma has risen in the last few years, because of the increased use of sexual aids and the more overt expression and possibilities of sadomasochistic sexual practices. These patients are not unstable. Trauma can follow anal intercourse using mechanical instruments, penile rings, or insertion of the whole forearm into the rectum. The reason for suspecting trauma is that the anal, rectal, and penile lesions tend to be atypical and unlike infective causes of ulceration, balanitis, etc. The lesions usually heal spontaneously but occasionally surgical repair is required.

Lymphocele

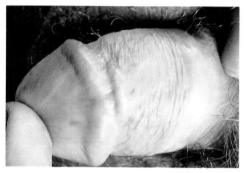

Lymphocele is a totally benign condition but very alarming to patients. The patient notices a cord-like swelling around the coroneal sulcus. It is sometimes accompanied by lymphangitis of the dorsum of the shaft. This may follow prolonged or particularly energetic sexual intercourse or masturbation, but this is by no means an essential prerequisite. The condition arises as a result of temporary obstruction of the lymphatics. No treatment is required, apart from reassurance and the explanation that it will resolve itself, which it does within a few days.

Peyronie's disease

- Aetiology unknown
- Pain and bending of penis
- Spontaneous resolution
- Surgery

Peyronie's disease is an alarming and distressing condition in which the patient first notices pain and permanent bending of the penis, particularly when erect. This is due to chronic fibrosis of the intercavernous septums of the penis. The condition may occur in association with Dupuytren's contracture. The aetiology is unknown. It usually occurs in middle aged men. On examination a hard ridge or lump of fibrous tissue may be felt on the dorsal aspect of the shaft of the penis and occasionally on the ventral and lateral aspect.

A few cases resolve spontaneously, which makes treatment claims difficult to assess. Surgical excision of the plaques is sometimes recommended.

Psychological effects

Doctors treating patients with disfiguring lesions of the genitals should not forget the profound psychological sequelae that may be associated with them. Patients often do not show their concern and practitioners may need to take the initiative in discussing these aspects and giving reassurance. If this is not possible or the condition is permanent psychiatric support may be needed.

SYPHILIS: CLINICAL FEATURES

Extent of the problem

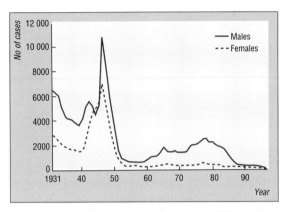

New cases of infectious syphilis seen in GUM clinics in England and Wales: 1931–96. Reproduced with permission from the PHLS Communicable Disease Surveillance Centre *The Communicable Disease Report* 1997;**7**:22.

The advent of penicillin made a dramatic and rapid impact on the incidence of early infectious syphilis throughout the world in the late 1940s. The number of cases of syphilis seen in clinics in England and Wales has declined substantially since the peak after the Second World War (27761). Latest figures (1996) indicate just over 1200 cases seen in clinics. Cases of infectious syphilis did show an increase in the 1960s and 1970s and began to fall in the late 1980s and early 1990s. It is thought that the rise probably indicated increasing transmission between men, and that the subsequent decline indicated a change in behaviour among homosexual men. Elsewhere in the world, syphilis still presents a major clinical problem and the World Health Organisation estimates that there are 12 million new cases of infectious syphilis worldwide each year, the majority of these cases occurring in South and South-East Asia (5.8 million), and Sub-Saharan Africa (3.5 million). In other countries such as the United States and Russia, syphilis is still a substantial problem. In the United States there was a major increase in infectious syphilis during the 1990s which is now declining but is still high, with rates among black-skinned people more than 40 times higher than those in white-skinned people. Currently in Russia and the Baltic states there is a major epidemic of infectious syphilis which started in the late 1980s.

Classification

Time after exposure

	Early infectious
9–90 days	Primary
6 weeks–6 months	Secondary
(4–8 weeks after primary lesion)	
2 years	Latent (early)
	Late non-infectious
≥2 years	Latent (late)
3–20 years	Neurosyphilis
	Cardiovascular syphilis
	Gummatous syphilis

Acquired syphilis has been classified traditionally into early infectious and late non-infectious stages. The arbitrary cut off point between these is usually two years.

Primary syphilis—The incubation period for primary syphilis is 9 to 90 days (mean 21 days). Lesions appear at the site of inoculation; these sites may sometimes be extragenital. The lesion is normally solitary and painless. It first appears as a red macule which progresses into a papule and finally ulcerates. This ulcer is usually round and clean with an indurated base and edges. Inguinal lymph nodes are moderately enlarged, rubbery, painless, and discrete. The primary lesions will heal within three to 10 weeks and may go unnoticed by the patient. Lesions on the cervix, rectum, anal canal, and margin may in particular be asymptomatic.

Secondary syphilis—The lesions of secondary syphilis usually occur four to eight weeks after the appearance of the primary lesion. In about one third of cases the primary lesion is still present. The lesions are generalised, affecting skin and mucous membranes.

The skin lesions are usually symmetrical and non-itchy. They can be macular, papular, papulosquamous, and very rarely pustular. The *macular* lesions (0·5–1 cm in diameter) on the shoulders, chest, back, abdomen, and arms. The *papular* lesions are coppery red and the same size as the macules. They may occur on the trunk, palms, arms, legs, soles, face, and genitalia. (Skin lesions are commonly a mixture of macular and papular (maculopapular).)

Sites of primary syphilis

Genital	*Extragenital*
Shaft of penis	Lip
Coronal sulcus	Tongue
Glans penis	Mouth, tonsil, pharynx
Prepuce	Fingers
Fraenum	Eyelid
Urethral meatus	Nipple
Anal margin/canal	Any part of skin or
Rectum	mucous membranes
Labia minora/majora	
Fourchette	
Clitoris	
Vaginal wall	
Cervix	

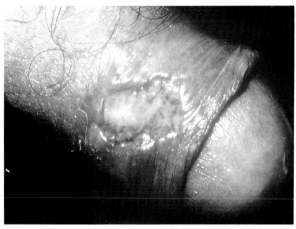
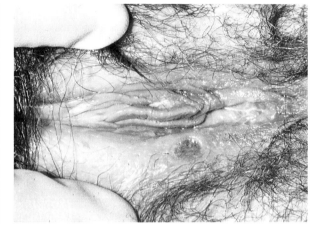

Primary chancre of penis and vulva

Lesions of secondary syphilis

Skin	Macular Papular	maculopapular
	Condylomata lata	
	Papulosquamous	
	Pustular	
Mucous membranes:	Erosions	

Clinical features of secondary syphilis

Skin lesions	75–80%
Mucous membrane lesions	30%
Generalised lymphadenopathy	50–60%
Arthritis, arthralgia, periostitis	
Hepatitis	
Glomerulonephritis and nephrotic syndrome	Rare
Iridocyclitis and choroidoretinitis	(<10%)
Neurological disease (meningitis, cranial nerve palsies)	
Alopecia	

In warm opposed areas of the body (anus, labia) papular lesions can become large and coalesce to appear as large fleshy masses (condylomata lata). The *papulosquamous* lesions are found when scaling of the papules occurs and can be seen in association with straightforward papular lesions. If papulosquamous lesions occur on the palms or soles they are sometimes described as psoriasiform. *Pustular* lesions are rare and occur when the papular lesions undergo central necrosis. *Mucous membrane* lesions are shallow, painless erosions which usually appear in association with papular skin lesions and affect the mucous surface of lips, cheeks, tongue, fauces, pharynx and larynx, nose, vulva, vagina, glans penis, prepuce, and cervix. They have a greyish appearance and are sometimes described as "snail track" ulcers.

The lesions of skin and mucous membrane may be associated with non-specific constitutional symptoms of malaise, fever, anorexia, and generalised lymphadenopathy. The secondary stage is one of bacteriaemia, and any organ may show evidence of this—for example, hepatitis, iritis, meningitis, and optic neuritis with papilloedema.

Features of secondary syphilis: maculopapular rash on hands and chest and condylomata lata

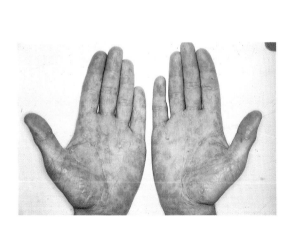
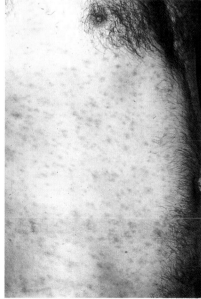
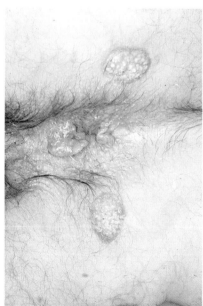

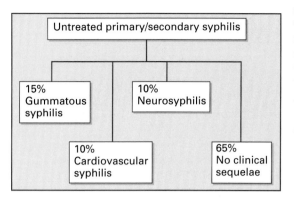

Latent syphilis—The latent period of syphilis follows the secondary stage. This latent period is divided into early and late. Early means that the disease has been present for less than two years and late for more than this time. The term latent means that there are no overt symptoms or signs of the disease and that the patient has never been treated. The condition is diagnosed from positive results to serological tests; no clinical evidence of early or late syphilis in any system; normal results on chest radiography and screening; and examination of cerebrospinal fluid to exclude cardiovascular syphilis or neurosyphilis. (Diagnosing syphilis is discussed in the next chapter.)

About 65% of patients with untreated syphilis will not develop late clinical sequelae of the disease. About 10% will develop neurological, 10% cardiovascular, and 15% gummatous lesions. It is extremely rare to see late syphilis any longer in the developed world, as a result of the decline in infectious syphilis and improved treatment and clinic facilities.

Neurosyphilis

Classification

- Asymptomatic
- Meningovascular
- Parenchymatous
  General paralysis of the insane
  Tabes dorsalis

Neurosyphilis is classified into asymptomatic, meningovascular, and parenchymatous (general paralysis of the insane and tabes dorsalis). The widespread use of antibiotics for other unrelated conditions has probably resulted in neurosyphilis which does not always fit the older classical clinical forms and descriptions.

Asymptomatic—As the name suggests, there are no neurological symptoms or signs and the diagnosis is based entirely on changes in the cerebrospinal fluid and serum.

Meningovascular disease can present at both early and late stages of syphilis. Patients can present with acute meningeal involvement during the secondary stages of the disease, often coinciding with the development of skin lesions. Headache is the main symptom. Signs of meningitis are found with third, sixth, and eighth cranial nerve involvement, papilloedema, and, rarely, homonymous hemianopia or hemiplegia. Late meningovascular syphilis presents less acutely but headaches may still be a presenting symptom. Cranial nerve palsies (third, sixth, seventh, and eighth) and pupillary abnormalities are seen. The pupils are small and unequal in size and react to accommodation but not light (Argyll Robertson pupils). Cerebral and spinal cord (anterior spinal artery) vessels may be affected. Epilepsy, confusion, aphasia, monoplegia, hemiplegia, or paraplegia, are just some of the ways in which late meningovascular syphilis can present.

Parenchymatous neurosyphilis may present as general paralysis of the insane, tabes dorsalis, or, rarely, a combination of the two. General paralysis with resulting cerebral atrophy 10–20 years after the original primary infection. Manifestations of the disease are a poor memory, lack of judgment and insight, delusions, confusion and mood swings, and sometimes convulsions. The signs can include a fine tremor of the lips, tongue, and hands; dysarthria; occasionally Argyll Robertson pupils and optic atrophy; hyperactive tendon reflexes; and extensor plantar responses (due to lesions of the pyramidal tract). Late in the disease the patient may suffer from dementia, a spastic paraplegia, and urinary and faecal incontinence.

General paralysis of the insane

Symptoms

Early	Late
Irritability	Defective judgment
Fatigability	Lack of insight
Inefficiency	Depression or euphoria
Personality changes	Confusion and disorientation
Headaches	
	Delusions
Impaired memory	
	Seizures
Tremors	
	Transient paralysis and aphasia

Signs

Expressionless facies

Tremor of lips, tongue, and hands

Dysarthria

Impairment of handwriting

Hyperactive tendon reflexes

Pupillary abnormalities

Optic atrophy

Convulsions

Extensor plantar responses

Tabes dorsalis is characterised by increasing ataxia, failing vision, sphincter disturbances, and attacks of severe pains. These pains are described as "lightning" since they occur as acute stabbing pain commonly in the legs. Attacks are fleeting or last a few days and classically occur at right angles to the limb. Paraesthesiae, incontinence, impotence, and tabetic crises may occur. These crises usually occur acutely and affect the stomach, rectum, bladder, urethra, kidneys, and larynx. The gastric crisis is the most common and the symptoms of epigastric pain and vomiting can be mistaken for an acute surgical abdomen.

Tabes dorsalis

Symptoms	Signs
Lightning pains	Argyll Robertson pupils
Ataxia	Absent ankle reflexes
Bladder disturbance	Absent knee reflexes
Paraesthesiae	Absent biceps and triceps reflexes
Tabetic crises	
Visual loss	Romberg's sign
Rectal incontinence	Impaired vibration sense
Deafness	Impaired position sense
Impotence	Impaired sense of touch and pain
	Optic atrophy
	Ocular palsies
	Charcot's joints

The signs of tabes dorsalis are largely due to degeneration of the posterior columns: absent ankle and knee reflexes (rarely biceps and triceps), impaired vibration and position sense, and a positive Romberg's sign. Argyll Robertson pupils are found in half of the cases and optic atrophy in a fifth. Charcot's arthropathy is rare, found in fewer than 10% of cases. The joints (knee, hip, ankle, spine, feet) are grossly disorganised and hypermobile with osteophyte formation and loose bodies in the joint. Finally, perforating ulcers of the feet can be found.

Cardiovascular syphilis

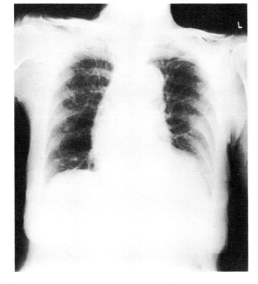

Cardiovascular syphilis most commonly occurs in large vessels, but medium and small sized ones may also be affected. The aorta is affected by an aortitis (with or without coronary ostial stenosis), an aneurysm of the ascending part, and aortic incompetence. Aneurysms of innominate, carotid, and subclavian vessels have also been described. Early changes are symptomless. Advancing aortitis may result in dull substernal pain or angina whereas aortic incompetence can present with acute left ventricular failure, paroxysmal nocturnal dyspnoea, and angina. The symptoms of aortic aneurysm vary depending on site; if in the ascending part (the commonest site) there may be dull substernal pain or angina and left ventricular failure. The symptoms of an aneurysm affecting the arch usually result from the pressure on structures within the superior mediastinum. Thus, stridor and cough (trachea), dysphagia (oesophagus), breathlessness (left bronchus), hoarseness (left recurrent laryngeal nerve), and Horner's syndrome (sympathetic chain) may occur. Finally, pressure on the superior vena cava can result in congested veins in the head and neck and cyanosis. The signs of cardiovascular disease are no different from those of aortic incompetence and aneurysms from other causes.

Gummatous syphilis

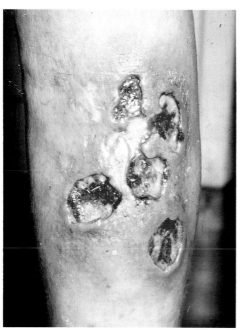

Gummas are granulamatous lesions appearing three to 12 years after the primary infection. Gummas may occur on the skin or mucous membranes and in bone or viscera. Skin lesions are usually modular. They can occur anywhere on the skin and appear as small groups of painless lesions which are indolent, firm, coppery red, and about 0·5–1 cm diameter. If subcutaneous tissue is affected the lesions start as smooth hard swellings which eventually break down into well circumscribed punched out ulcers which, when they heal, leave typical tissue paper scarring. These occur on the leg, face, and scalp. Lesions in mucous membrane appear as punched out ulcers on the hard and soft palate, uvula, tongue, larynx, pharynx, and nasal septum. Bone and visceral gummas are extremely rare, affecting the tibia, skull, clavicle, sternum, femur, liver, brain, oesophagus, stomach, lung, and testes.

SYPHILIS: DIAGNOSIS AND MANAGEMENT

- History
- Physical examination
  ±
- Dark ground microscopy
- Serology
- Lumbar puncture
- Chest radiography and screening

Establishing a diagnosis of syphilis, whatever the stage of the disease, can be difficult and it is wise for all suspected cases to be referred for specialised tests and management in a department of genitourinary medicine. The diagnosis can be confirmed by the history, physical examination, and one or all of four tests—dark ground microscopy, serology, examination of cerebrospinal fluid, and radiology. Which of these tests appear as positive will depend on the clinical stage of the patient's syphilis.

Dark ground microscopy

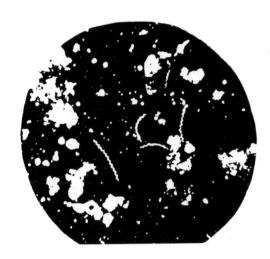

Dark ground microscopy can be used to establish the diagnosis from the lesions of primary and secondary syphilis or occasionally from material obtained by puncture of inguinal nodes (after recent topical application of antiseptic or antibiotic or when lesions are healed or concealed). The presence of oral commensal treponemes makes microscopy unreliable for mouth lesions. Three separate specimens from the lesion(s) should be examined by dark ground microscopy initially and, if necessary, on three consecutive days. This is done by cleaning the lesion with a gauze swab soaked in normal saline and squeezing it to encourage a serum exudate. The serum is then scraped off the lesion and placed on the three slides. After a cover slip has been placed on the material microscopy can be performed. Dark ground microscopy is a vital test since in primary syphilis it may be the only positive means of establishing the diagnosis. Considerable experience is required to recognise *Treponema pallidum*. It is bluish white, closely coiled (8–24), and 6–20 μm long. There are three characteristic movements of the treponeme: watch spring, corkscrew, and angular. Serological tests for syphilis are not always positive when primary lesions occur; the tests do not give positive results until about two weeks after the appearance of the chancre, about three to five weeks after infection.

Serological tests

Non-specific tests
- Venereal Disease Research Laboratory test
- Rapid plasma reagin test
- Wassermann reaction

Specific tests
- Absorbed fluorescent treponemal antibody test
- *Treponema pallidum* haemagglutination test

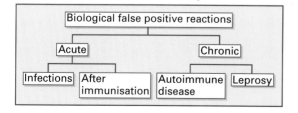

The serological tests used in the diagnosis of syphilis are either non-specific or specific.

Non-specific tests—The most useful non-specific tests are either the Venereal Disease Research Laboratory test (VDRL) or the rapid plasma reagin (RPR) test which have now replaced the Wassermann reaction. Essentially these tests depend on the appearance of antibody (reagin) in the serum, and this may not occur until three to five weeks after the patient has contracted the infection. Thus the VDRL/RPR tests will give positive results in only about 75% of cases of primary syphilis. They are quantitative tests and this can be useful in assessing the stage and activity of the disease. The VDRL test is a flocculation test. Positive results may occur for three reasons. Firstly, technical errors may occur because of mistakes in collection, labelling, and reporting of specimens or the use of faulty materials. The moral is that the diagnosis of syphilis should never be made on the basis of only one set of tests. Secondly, positive results occur in syphilis and other treponemal conditions similar to syphilis (yaws, bejel, and pinta), but in such instances the specific tests will also be positive. Thirdly, there may be acute or chronic biological false positive reactions.

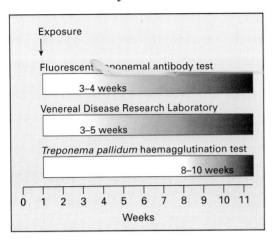

| | **Stage of disease** | | | |
	Primary %	Secondary %	Latent %	Late %
Venereal Disease Research Laboratory test	75	100	75	75
Treponema pallidum haemagglutination test	60	100	97	100
Fluorescent treponemal antibody test	90	100	97	100

Results positive	**Diagnosis**
None	Syphilis not present or very early primary syphilis
All	Untreated, recently treated, or latent syphilis
VDRL and FTA	Primary syphilis
TPHA and FTA	Treated syphilis or untreated latent or late
FTA only	Early primary syphilis—untreated or recently treated early syphilis
TPHA only	Treated syphilis
VDRL only	False positive reaction

Biological false positive reactions—The acute type of reaction is transient, lasting a few weeks to six months. Such reactions occur after viral infections (such as glandular fever, measles, chicken pox, mumps, herpes simplex and zoster, viral pneumonia) or after immunisation against typhoid and yellow fever. The chronic false positive reaction can last for many years or even a lifetime. It is seen particularly in autoimmune diseases (disseminated lupus erythematosis, haemolytic anaemia, thyroiditis) and rheumatoid arthritis. Sometimes the VDRL test is positive years before the patient develops one of these conditions. Specific tests for syphilis will be negative.

Specific tests—The two specific tests most often used to establish a diagnosis of treponemal disease are the absorbed fluorescent treponemal antibody test (FTA-ABS) and the *Treponema pallidum* haemagglutination (TPHA) test. The fluorescent treponemal antibody test is the first serological test (either specific or non-specific) to become positive; this usually occurs three to four weeks after infection. Thus this test is positive in 85–90% of cases of primary syphilis. In early untreated primary disease it may be the only positive serological test. (The FTA is not a routine screening test, therefore if early syphilis is suspected this test will need to be requested of the laboratory.) It must not be forgotten, however, that all serological tests may be negative despite the presence of a primary lesion. The *Treponema pallidum* haemagglutination test is the last of the serological tests to become positive. Thus it will always be positive in the secondary stages of disease but only so in 60% of patients presenting with primary syphilis. As already emphasised, these specific tests can distinguish only between treponemal and non-treponemal disease but not between the different treponemal conditions. Occasionally a clinical distinction can be made, for example, between syphilis and yaws.

The findings of positive serological tests for syphilis should not necessarily be interpreted as showing that the patient has active or untreated latent disease. Thus, for example, in patients who have received adequate treatment the VDRL test may still be positive (particularly if treated late on in the infection). Responses to the fluorescent treponemal antibody and *Treponema pallidum* haemagglutination tests often remain positive for life despite adequate treatment.

Syphilis has been controlled in the United Kingdom largely because of the policy of screening patients attending antenatal clinics, departments of genitourinary medicine, and blood transfusion centres and by selective use in neurological and psychiatric assessment of certain patients. Currently the best combination of tests for screening for treponemal disease is the VDRL or RPR test and the *Treponema pallidum* haemagglutination test.

Cerebrospinal fluid and radiology

Investigations of cerebrospinal fluid

- Cell count
- Total protein
- IgG estimation (or Lange colloidal gold curve)
- Venereal Disease Research Laboratory, *Treponema pallidum* haemagglutination, and fluorescent treponemal antibody tests

Abnormalities of the cerebrospinal fluid may be found at any stage of syphilis and may occur early (primary and secondary stages) without symptoms. Lumbar puncture may be necessary to exclude neurosyphilis or as part of the investigation of any patient with suspected latent disease. This investigation should be carried out if the patient has neurological symptoms or signs. The following tests can be performed on cerebrospinal fluid: cell count, total protein, IgG estimation, or Lange colloidal gold curve (no longer used widely), and the three serological tests. The findings vary according to the type of neurosyphilis. A cell count above 0.005×10^9 lymphocytes per litre and protein above 40 g/l would be considered abnormal. The VDRL test on the fluid is unreliable in diagnosing neurosyphilis since it is negative in up to half of all patients with active neurosyphilis. A positive fluorescent treponemal antibody or *Treponema pallidum*

Changes in cerebrospinal fluid in neurosyphilis

	Stage of disease				
	Asymptomatic	Meningo-vascular		Parenchy-matous	
		Early	Late	General paralysis of the insane	Tabes dorsalis
Cell count	±	+++	++	++	+
Protein	+	++	++	++	+
FTA	+	+	+	+	+/−
VDRL	−	+	±	++	+/−
TPHA	+	+	+	+	+/−
Pressure	Normal	++	±	Normal	Normal

haemagglutination test result, or both, can result from a transudate of IgG specific for *Treponema pallidum* in patients whose disease has been adequately treated. It therefore does not indicate active disease of the nervous system; negative results, however, virtually rule out neurosyphilis.

The final diagnostic procedure in the assessment of a patient with latent disease or cardiovascular disease is a chest radiograph (posteroanterior, left lateral) to show the arch of the aorta and screening to detect aortic dilatation. More specialised tests may subsequently be indicated.

Treatment and prognosis

Herxheimer reaction

	% Of patients affected
Primary	50%
Secondary	70–90%
Early latent	25%
Late latent	20%
Neurosyphillis { general paralysis	50–75%
tabes	Rare
Cardiovascular	Rare

Penicillin remains the cornerstone of the treatment of all types of syphilis. In primary and secondary syphilis aqueous procaine penicillin should be given for 10 days. Successful treatment depends on obtaining a minimum serum concentration of 30 IU/l and maintaining this over a long period. If there is any anxiety about patients returning or if they cannot attend daily, erythromycin or tetracycline/doxycycline (except for neurosyphilis) can be substituted. Also these can be used in patients allergic to penicillin. Since the cure rate is lower with these, many physicians will repeat treatment after three months.

The Jarisch–Herxheimer reaction is common in primary and secondary syphilis and patients must be warned that fever and flu-like symptoms may occur 3–12 hours after the first injection; occasionally the chancre or skin lesions enlarge or become more widespread. Aspirin is recommended.

Other stages or manifestations of syphilis are also treated with procaine penicillin. Steroids, to eliminate the Herxheimer reaction, are used only in patients with neurosyphilis or cardiovascular syphilis who may develop focal lesions (cerebrovascular or coronary artery occlusion) and mania, confusion, and psychosis.

The prognosis of treated syphilis depends on the stage of the disease and degree of tissue damage in the cardiovascular and neurological systems. Thus adequate treatment of primary, secondary, and latent stages and asymptomatic neurosyphilis will result in cure and halt progression of the disease. The prognosis in symptomatic cardiovascular and neurosyphilis is variable. In general the inflammatory process is arrested by adequate treatment but the tissue damage may be too great to prevent an improvement in symptoms.

Contact tracing must be carried out on all sexual contacts that a patient with early infectious syphilis has had in the preceding three to six months. In late syphilis, when the patient is no longer infectious, serological testing is probably only practicable in the patient's regular partner. If late syphilis is diagnosed in a mother it may by necessary to test her children. Syphilis during pregnancy is discussed in the next chapter. Syphilis is a complex disease and its diagnosis, management, and follow up should not be undertaken by the non-specialist.

The illustration of dark ground microscopy was taken from King A, Nicoll C, and Rodin P, *Veneral Diseases*, published by Ballière Tindall.

Treatment of syphilis

Stage	Standard treatment	Alternatives		Prognosis
Primary and secondary	Aqueous procaine penicillin* 600 000 units/day 10 days	**If penicillin allergy:** Erythromycin ⎫ 500 mg four times Tetracycline ⎬ a day 14 days Doxycycline — 100 mg twice a day for 14 days		Excellent Relapse exceptionally first year
Latent: early (≤ 2 years duration)	Aqueous procaine penicillin* 600 000 units/day 10 days	**If patient unable to attend daily:** Benzathine penicillin 2·4 MU once only		
late (> 2 years)	Aqueous procaine penicillin* 900 000 units/day 21 days	**If penicillin allergy or unable to attend daily:** Erythromycin ⎫ 500 mg four times Tetracycline ⎬ a day 30 days Doxycycline — 100 mg twice a day for 14 days		Excellent
Neurosyphilis and cardiovascular syphilis	Aqueous procaine penicillin* 900 000 units/day 21 days + prednisone 5 mg four times daily for one day before penicillin, and then same dose for two days after	**If penicillin allergy confirm that real penicillin allergy and consider desensitisation:** Oxytetracycline 500 mg four times a day 30 days Doxycycline 100 mg twice daily 30 days	Not suitable for neuro-syphilis	Depends on type of neurosyphilis and extent of cardiovascular disease
Gummatous	Aqueous procaine penicillin* 600 000 units/day 15 days	**If penicillin allergy:** Erythromycin ⎫ 500 mg four times Tetracycline ⎬ a day for 15 days		

* When procaine penicillin is used protenecid 500 mg twice a day given for same time interval

PREGNANCY AND THE NEONATE

- Herpes
- Chlamydia
- Gonorrhoea
- Syphilis
- Cytomegalovirus

The consequences of sexually transmitted diseases for the unborn or newly born child are extremely emotive, when they need not be so. Most of the maternal diseases that can affect the fetus or neonate can be prevented or are usually not serious if recognised and treated early. The unpreventable or unprevented diseases, however, although rare, may have serious and lifelong consequences.

Genital herpes

Risk of neonatal herpes

- Primary attack in mother in third trimester or at delivery 40–50%
- Recurrent attack in mother at delivery 0–8%

There are two problems associated with infection with genital herpes simplex virus during pregnancy: congenital infection and neonatal infection. It is theoretically possible for transplacental transmission to occur but evidence for this is poor. If it does occur it is likely to result in fetal death and spontaneous abortion. Neonatal herpes is a very rare disease in the United Kingdom with recognised infection occurring in only 1·6/100,000 livebirths. Higher rates of neonatal infection are reported from the United States and other parts of Europe. Neonatal infection can occur if the mother has active herpes at the time of delivery, either with lesions or without (asymptomatic viral shedding). The risk to the neonate is greater from primary than from recurrent episodes in the mother.

Over 95% of infected babies are born to women who are unaware that they have genital herpes. These women may be shedding virus asymptomatically, or the infant may acquire the infection after delivery from maternal labial herpes or herpes infection in one of the medical or nursing staff or other babies.

Neonatal herpes, although rare, can be fatal within the first few weeks or result in permanent brain damage in the survivors. The disease can present either in a localised or disseminated form. The overall mortality is about 60%.

Women with genital herpes who become pregnant are understandably concerned about the risk of transmitting infection to their babies.

Sources of neonatal herpes infection

- Mother—labial, cervical, vulval lesions
- Medical and nursing staff, other babies/relatives

Management

As the majority of babies with neonatal herpes are born to women without a history of genital herpes, all pregnant women should be examined at the onset of labour for signs of infection and then managed in accordance with the recommendations below.

Women with a history of recurrent genital herpes who seek advice on the management of herpes in pregnancy often get conflicting advice on how their infection should be managed. They can be reassured that their risk of transmitting herpes to their baby is low. It is not possible to predict which women will transmit infection by taking viral cultures during late gestation and these are therefore *not* indicated. There is also no indication for caesarean section in women who do not have genital lesions at delivery. Symptomatic recurrences of genital herpes during pregnancy will not harm the fetus. Vaginal delivery is appropriate if no lesions are present at delivery. Current practice in the United Kingdom is for delivery by caesarean section in women who have a lesional recurrence at term; however the risks of vaginal delivery for the fetus are small and must be set against risks to the mother of caesarean section.

In contrast women who have their first episode of genital herpes during pregnancy are at much greater risk of transmitting the virus, particularly if they acquire infection during the third trimester. A woman infected during the first or second trimester should be managed in line with her clinical condition. This will often involve the use of either oral or intravenous acyclovir in standard doses.

Sequelae of neonatal infection without treatment

	Mortality	Serious impairment of survivors
Skin, eye, mouth	Rare	Up to 30%
Encephalitis	50%	50%
Disseminated	80%	Most

Providing that delivery does not ensue, the pregnancy should be managed expectantly and vaginal delivery anticipated. Continuous acyclovir in the last four weeks of pregnancy may prevent recurrence at term and hence the need for delivery by caesarean section. Caesarean section should be considered for all women who acquire infection in the third trimester, particularly those developing symptoms within six weeks of delivery as the risk of viral shedding in labour is very high. If vaginal delivery is unavoidable, acyclovir treatment of mother and baby may be indicated.

While prevention of infection during pregnancy is obviously important, research evidence on how best to do this is lacking. Pregnant women whose partners have genital herpes should be strongly advised not to have sex when he is symptomatic. Condom use throughout pregnancy may reduce the risk of transmission.

Chlamydial infections

Conjunctivitis	Pneumonia
Otitis media	Failure to thrive
Nasopharyngitis	

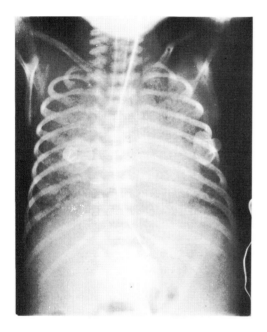

Chlamydia trachomatis can be transmitted by direct inoculation into the neonate's eye or by inhalation of infected material during birth; 30–50% of infants born to infected mothers will develop eye disease and 10–20% a pneumonia. The eye disease appears one to three weeks after birth and varies from a mild inclusion conjunctivitis to a purulent and severe ophthalmia with oedema of the eyelids and palpebral conjunctiva. In half of all cases the condition is a bilateral. If untreated the condition usually resolves spontaneously, but in rare instances it can progress to conjunctival scarring and micropannus formation.

A nasopharyngitis or pneumonia, resulting from the inhalation of infected material at birth, usually presents one to three months after birth. The infant with pneumonia is usually afebrile with a paroxysmal staccato cough, tachypnoea, occasionally apnoea, and sometimes an associated nasal discharge and otitis media. There is failure to thrive in most cases. The chest radiograph shows hyperexpansion with bilaterial symmetrical diffuse interstitial and patchy alveolar infiltrates. About half the infants also have conjunctivitis or a history of it.

Diagnosis—Eye, nasopharyngeal, or lung disease due to chlamydia is diagnosed by isolating the organism. The pneumonia is usually associated with eosinophilia, raised serum IgG and IgM concentrations, and raised titres to *C trachomatis*.

Treatment—Chlamydial conjunctivitis should be treated systemically since up to half the infants may later develop a nasopharyngitis or pneumonia. Application of ointment into the eye is difficult and unnecessary. Saline bathing can be used. Erythromycin ethylsuccinate should be used in divided doses up to a total of 50 mg/kg body weight/day for 10–14 days. The pneumonia should be treated with the same regimen.

Both the mother and father should be examined to look for *C trachomatis* and any other concurrent sexually acquired condition.

Gonococcal infections

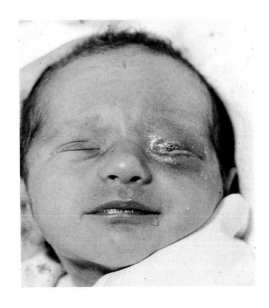

Gonococcal conjunctivitis is transmitted in the same way as chlamydial infection. The inflammation and purulent discharge are usually evident within a few days of birth. Rarely colonisation of the pharynx and rectum and a gonococcal septicaemia (similar to that found in adults) can be seen.

Diagnosis is by microscopy and culture of infected material from the eye. Systemic treatment is required. As with chlamydial ophthalmia local insertion of antibiotic into the eye is not sufficient or necessary but saline bathing may be applied. Systemic penicillin is required. Ceftriaxone can be used, for example 25–50 mg/kg IV or IM in a single dose, not to exceed 125 mg. The mother and her sexual contacts will also require investigation and, if necessary, treatment.

Ophthalmia neonatorum (a conjunctivitis within 21 days of birth) is notifiable. A chlamydial or gonococcal infection should always be suspected in an infant with a sticky eye, and these two organisms should be excluded in every case. These conditions are not the commonest causes of a sticky eye in neonates but the increasing incidence of chlamydial infections now makes this form of ophthalmia five times more common than gonococcal.

Syphilis

Treatment of mother with syphilis during pregnancy	
Early infectious syphilis	Procaine penicillin 600 000 units intramuscularly daily for 10 days
Other stages	Same as in non-pregnant state
If allergic to penicillin	Erythromycin

Unlike infections with herpes, chlamydia, and gonorrhoea, which are acquired at birth, syphilis is a prenatal infection. Fetal infection may occur at any time during pregnancy. It is more likely to occur if the mother has primary, secondary, or early latent syphilis since considerable numbers of organisms are present in the circulation during these stages. The infectivity when the mother has untreated primary or secondary disease is virtually 100%. This decreases the longer the mother has been suffering from her disease. It is uncommon for a woman with late syphilis to give birth to a child with congenital disease but it is possible, even though previous pregnancies may have been normal.

Congenital syphilis is no longer a public health problem in developed countries. The low incidence of congenital syphilis in the United Kingdom (two cases in 1996) is due largely to the control of early acquired infectious syphilis in women and through screening all pregnant women for syphilis. The World Health Organisation estimates that there are 12 million new cases of infectious syphilis worldwide each year. The largest number of new cases are found in South and South-East Asia (5.8 million) and Sub-Saharan Africa (3.5 million).

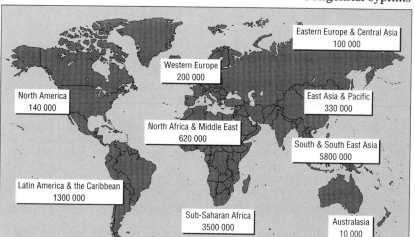

Annual global incidence of new cases of syphilis: estimated numbers and geographical distribution in people aged 15–49 years (estimated total 12 million cases)

Serological tests should be carried out at the first antenatal visit. It is still possible for the mother to become infected after this or for her to be incubating the disease with negative serological results. Women at high risk of infection should therefore have the tests repeated in the final trimester.

A pregnant woman found to have syphilis is likely to be suffering from early infectious syphilis. If so the appropriate treatment is aqueous procaine penicillin 600 000 units intramuscularly daily for 10 days. Other stages of syphilis require the same treatment as used in the non-pregnant patient (see previous chapter). Penicillin given during pregnancy produces a prevention and cure rate of virtually 100%. If the mother is allergic to penicillin, erythromycin (not the estolate) can be used at a level of 500 mg six hourly for 15 days, or for 30 days if she has latent infection. Placental transfer of this drug can be inadequate, so it does not reliably cure an infected fetus. Therefore it is essential to be absolutely certain that the patient has a genuine sensitivity to penicillin, and to consider desensitisation. If penicillin cannot be used for the mother, the baby should have a course of penicillin at birth as a precaution.

Even if the mother has had an adequate course of penicillin during pregnancy the baby should be examined and serological tests carried out. Despite treatment of the mother, her serological results may still be positive at term. As passive transfer of antibody from the mother to the baby can occur, time must be allowed for this carryover to disappear (at least six weeks). Thus tests are carried out on the baby at six weeks and three months after birth.

There is some debate whether treatment in subsequent pregnancies is indicated. Some clinicians believe that this is desirable because of the possible persistence of the treponeme in the body after treatment and subsequent transplacental transfer. If the mother has been followed up for two years after treatment and discharged as cured an alternative approach is not to treat her in subsequent pregnancies but to perform serological tests for syphilis on the baby at the age of 3 months.

Congenital syphilis

When it occurs, congenital syphilis is classified into early, latent, and late stages. The clinical picture varies depending on the stage. The lesions of late syphilis can appear at varying intervals during the child's life.

Clinical features of congenital syphilis	
Early	Similar to adult secondary disease: rash, mucous membrane lesions, lymphadenopathy, ±lesions of bone, viscera, eye, central nervous system
Latent (early and late)	No clinical signs of active disease ± stigmata. Positive serological test results
Late (≥2)	Similar to adult late disease. Interstitial keratitis, osteoperiostitis, joint effusions, usually knees (Clutton's joints). Gumma hard and soft palate, pharynx. 8th Nerve deafness. Neurological features. Cardiovascular complications. Stigmata

The lesions of early and late congenital syphilis may heal but leave stigmata. On the *face and mouth* a saddle nose deformity and collapse of the bridge of the nose may occur as a result of rhinitis and gumma of the nasal septum. The face may look flat owing to impaired development of maxillae, and frontal bossing (Parrot's nodes) can be seen. Linear scars (rhagades) around the angles of the mouth result from healed mucocutaneous lesions of early disease. In the *teeth* the upper central incisors are smaller than normal and peg or barrel shaped and have a classically notched centre (Hutchinson's incisors). The molars can also be affected and show a rounded appearance (Moon's molars). In the *eyes* scarring can remain as a result of earlier choroidal involvement and opacities of the cornea and ghost vessels can be seen as a result of interstitial keratitis. *Bone lesions* include sabre tibia following previous osteoperiostitis.

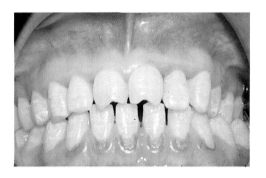

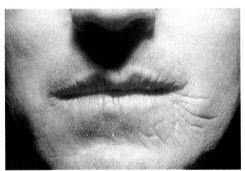

Early congenital syphilis—The clinical picture may arouse suspicion, but confirmatory tests are required. Clinical manifestations may present only after several weeks. Dark field microscopy from skin lesions or nasal discharge can establish the diagnosis immediately. Positive serological findings are confirmatory. Serological tests for syphilis (Venereal Diseases Research Laboratory and *Treponema pallidum* haemagglutination tests) should be performed at birth, but passive transfer from the mother will make interpretation of these impossible early on, and they should be repeated at 6 and 12 weeks. A rising titre is compatible with congenital disease. In the last few years the fluorescent treponemal antibody absorbed IgM test has been used in an attempt to differentiate passive transfer from true congenital disease at an early stage. Specific IgM in the neonate has been thought to indicate congenital disease; unfortunately false positive and negative results do occur and it is probably not wise to rely on this test for such an important diagnosis. In the presence of positive results to standard serological tests (Venereal Diseases Research Laboratory and *Treponema pallidum* haemagglutination tests) there is no substitute for waiting a number of weeks. The baby will not suffer from delay in treatment, but the parents may, of course, be anxious. Their anxiety has to be weighed against making an early diagnosis that may be wrong, and labelling the baby with the diagnosis of congenital syphilis for the rest of its life, making the parents guilty about the disease that they have passed on.

Latent and late congenital syphilis—Most cases of latent and late syphilis are identified because of incidental serological tests for syphilis. Sometimes cases are found when the patient or parent consults because of impairment of hearing (nerve deafness) or sight, swollen knee (Clutton's joints), or because other gross stigmata of disease are present. Serological tests will invariably give positive results. Other features, such as old interstitial keratitis and ghost vessels, should be looked for by slit lamp examination.

Early and late congenital syphilis—The treatment in early congenital syphilis is intramuscular procaine penicillin 50 000 units/kg body weight IM a day for 10–14 days. In late congenital syphilis the treatment is as for the equivalent stage in late acquired adult syphilis. The daily dose for children or adolescents is adjusted according to weight.

The illustration of gonococcal opthalmia was taken from King A, Nicoll C, and Rodin P, *Venereal Diseases*, published by Ballière Tindall.

PSYCHOLOGICAL AND SEXUAL PROBLEMS

DAVID GOLDMEIER

Sexual norms, psychological and sexual problems

Some sexual norms

Mean age at coitarche (years)	17 (1990)
	21 (1955)
Prevelence of anal sex in women	13%
Homosexual experiences (male and female)	
Ever (includes bisexuals)	5%
Exclusively homosexual	1–2%
Mean length of erect penis	5·25 inch
Penis deviates to left or right on erection	15%
Penis deviates up or down on erection	20%

Small penises (non-erect) increase in size significantly more than large penises on erection

Women can have as many as five to six orgasms in a few minutes

Breast size may increase by up to 25% during sexual arousal and orgasm

Mean heterosexual frequency of intercourse in the United Kingdom is four times a month

Rates of intercourse in a couple decrease after the "honeymoon period" (say 3–6 months)

The vaginal pH may be raised for up to three hours after sexual arousal

---

Psychosocial factors influencing whether sexual intercourse takes place or not

Factors	Explanation
Age	Libido decreases with age
Religion	Many religions have ethos of monogamy or celibacy and do not accept extramarital intercourse
Ethnic or cultural	Wife sharing in some cultures
Prostitution	Sexual contact certain unless prostitute discriminates against "high risk" clients
Illicit drugs or alcohol	May cause sexual disinhibition
Personality	Extroverts more likely to have casual intercourse
Sexual orientation	Before HIV homosexual men had high rate of partner change
"Infatuation"	"Falling in love" likely to lead to intercourse (biological? cultural?)
Unusual environment	Holidays or conferences—casual intercourse more likely
Psychiatric illness	Depression—decreased chance of intercourse Hypomania—increased chance of intercourse
Condom use (or non-use)	Inaccessability of, dislike or limited sexual pleasure with condoms. Trust in partner or partner already using non-barrier contraception

---

Apart from the diagnosis and treatment of STDs sexual health includes among other areas health that may pertain to contraception, termination of pregnancy, prevention of cervical cancer, and sexual dysfunction. All these can be construed as life events to the patient and consequently have greater or lesser psychological implications and sequelae.

Patients' complaints may reflect ignorance in one or more areas of genital anatomy and physiology, although young people receive much better sexual education than in former years.

Psychological factors are major influences determining whether or not sexual intercourse will take place. Once the patient knows he/she has an STD, or its presence is feared, the patient's emotions are difficult to dismiss.

Unless a patient has been raped (see below), acquisition of STD can be seen as the result of a more or less conscious decision taken before physical contact. Various factors influence patients in deciding whether or not intercourse should take place.

Most patients who attend STD clinics will talk relatively freely about sexual matters if the physician is sympathetic and empathic. With gentle coaxing they will also discuss their psychological problems given enough time.

HIV disease apart, psychological illness is clinically obvious in 1–2% of attenders at STD clinics and is detectable by validated questionnaire in up to 40% of patients.

Psychological and psychosexual problems encountered in a clinic may be classified into:

- Primary psychiatric disease states.
- Psychological disease secondary to sexually transmitted disease.
- Sexual, marital, relationship problems, and rape.

Most patients attending an STD clinic worry about having such an infection. If no disease is present, doctors must reassure

Classification of hypochondriasis

Psychiatric phenomenon	Description of phenomenon	Psychiatric illness/underlying phenomenon
Phobia	Fear of disease dispelled by discussion with doctor, but returns quickly	Anxiety, neurotic depression, obsessional illness
Delusion	Fixed false conviction of disease not altered by discussion	Monosymptomatic delusion, schizophrenia, psychotic depression

patients in clear simple language. If two sessions, say 10 to 15 minutes each, have not achieved this result, and the patient still believes he or she has an STD the patient may be said to have hypochondriasis. Hypochondriasis may be further classified symptomatically into phobias and delusions.

Phobias are best managed by cognitive behaviour therapy and/or selective serotonin reuptake inhibitors (SSRIs) or tricyclic antidepressants. Such psychiatric states may underlie sexual dysfunctions (see below).

Delusions should be managed by the psychitrists.

Psychological disease secondary to STD

Gonococcal and non-gonococcal urethritis

Gonorrhoea is usually easily and rapidly treated, and early intercourse after tests of cure in an otherwise stable relationship may help to heal the psychological wounds that one or both partners feel. Unfortunately non-gonococcal urethritis may be recurrent or even chronic in the absence of any detectable infection, and the man may have been told not to resume intercourse until the inflammation has subsided. It is mandatory that the physician treats the patient not his pus cells. Prolonged sexual abstinence may put a profound strain on the relationship, which is exacerbated if the female partner of a monogamous couple is told (incorrectly) to return at each spontaneous recurrence where there has been no sexual exposure outside the relationship. There is a lot to be said for seeing the couple together, so that their treatment can be coordinated and explained. The physician can also gauge the effects of and the necessity for sexual abstinence, can assess their relationship, and can facilitate discussion about the urethritis and possible underlying problems in the relationship.

Prostatic pain

Patients with prostatitis and prostatadynia are commonly anxious, and some are depressed. Pain thresholds decrease in the presence of anxiety. As well as antibiotic therapy where appropriate, explanation, reassurance, hypnotherapy, acupuncture, cognitive behaviour therapy, and antidepressant medication can all help to diminish the pain and make the patient feel more content.

Pelvic pain

Pelvic pain may be caused by pelvic inflammatory disease or by other conditions in the pelvis. Many patients with pelvic inflammatory disease complain of deep dyspareunia, and may also be infertile or subfertile. As well as dealing with the feelings of loss of health and fertility, the physician may usefully see the individual or the couple to pinpoint problems that have arisen out of one or both partners having had intercourse with others, and to discuss the resulting feelings of resentment and anger. Adequate sexual arousal ensures the cervix and uterus are lifted or "tented", so that penile buffeting is minimised.

Genital herpes

First-attack genital herpes is distressing not only because of the physical symptoms but also because of the grief reaction that can follow the realisation of a future with a chronic, painful, sometimes frequently recurring,

genital infection that can be passed on to the very people the person wants to cherish and protect. It can also tarnish the patient's personal and sexual self-esteem. However, these problems may have antedated the infection. Others who know about their illness may see them as at worst a pariah and at best the butt of jokes about herpes. Because of ignorance herpes may be understood synonymously with HIV infection. Unfortunately severe primary genital herpes may be followed by secondary vaginismus (see below).

There may be a positive association between non-coping patient personalities and frequency of recurrences. Non-psychotic psychiatric illness also possibly predicts frequent recurrences. The "stress" described by some patients before recurrences may be genuine anxiety or endogenous cytokine responses (eg interferon) to early virus replication. Patients with frequent recurrences need to be given the time and space to discuss their illness and their emotions. Physicians and psychologists in specially designated clinics for patients troubled by genital herpes attempt to alter their fear and negative self-image. This is important, because even with the use of continuous antivirals, a 100% reassurance can not be given that the infection cannot be passed on to others.

Simple education should not be forgotten. Patients with genital herpes incorrectly fear they will develop cervical cancer, become infertile and fatally infect their newborn babies (a rare event).

It is now possible technically to screen populations for the presence of serum herpes simplex type I and II antibodies. Most persons in the general population with type II antibodies deny that they have or do not know the significance of any genital lesions they might have. It is unknown at the present time exactly how to use such tests for the patients' benefit, but in some situations, for example an asymptomatic partner of a patient with frequent recurrences, a positive test result may come as a relief, whereas blanket screening without prior counselling may yield psychologically devastated patients where a positive result came "out of the blue".

Genital candidiasis

Frequent recurrences of genital candidiasis may leave both partners confused, frustrated and angry about the supposed source of the problem. A steady, stable relationship should be able to withstand this problem (which is not a "venereal disease") with the minimum of counselling. The finding of *Candida albicans* in genital secretions may tempt the physician to make an organic diagnosis, whereas the real problem may, for example, be vaginismus with the incidental finding of *C albicans*.

Trichomoniasis and bacterial vaginosis

Olfactory perception of sexual odours varies between the extremes of delusions of non-present smells, to denial of physically overwhelmingly repulsive discharges. In the usual clinical scenario, one or both partners can find the offensive vaginal discharges sexually offputting. After treatment, in spite of the absence of any objective smell, the woman may have lost confidence in her physiological body odour, and the man may mistake her normal musky exudate for the previous offensive discharge. The couple may need to be seen together, to hear the physician assure them of the normality of the discharge.

Syphilis

Syphilis is a special case, whether congenital or acquired. Many older patients would rather have a cancer than syphilis. This is not surprising considering that even in the 1950s two-thirds of inpatient psychiatric residents had tertiary syphilis. Similarly, congenital syphilis presenting in later life may devastate the patient with the realisation of his/her parents' infection and how it was acquired.

Genital warts

Apart from cervical carcinoma and dysplasia, genital warts are important to the patient for cosmetic reasons—both physical and psychological. What the patient is told about these otherwise trivial lesions can be important. It is now fashionable and probably legally required in many cases to tell patients their exact diagnosis and its implications. In many disease states immunological, physiological and clinical aspects of the illness may deteriorate when a catastrophic (though accurate) account of the disease is given. Thus in the case of genital warts saying "you have a potentially precancerous condition" to an anxious patient rather than "you have an infectious, cosmetically removable condition" is bad medicine and does not enhance the patient's recovery. A good physician always knows how and when to impart not such good news and always makes the patient feel better.

HIV disease

To a greater or lesser extent all patients with HIV disease have psychological problems. Many of the major risk groups for HIV infection have psychological problems prior to infection. Homosexual men may become anxious or depressed because of actual or feared non-acceptance of their sexuality by family, friends, or employers. Intravenous drug addicts have the multitude of problems that their illness brings, apart from the personality disorders that antedate the drug abuse.

All patients should be counselled before an HIV antibody test is undertaken, as important issues may need to be discussed.

Important psychological issues in counselling patients before an HIV test

(1) General facts about HIV disease
(2) Meanings of positive and negative tests
(3) Confidentiality of the results
(4) Handling stress and psychiatric illness in relation to taking the test
(5) Potential problems with insurance companies
(6) Social difficulties that may be encountered if result is positive

---

Social rejection by hostile family and friends and dismissal by employers and insurance companies must all be considered. Counselling may provoke very uncomfortable feelings, particularly when the patient has never really considered a positive result. Nowadays, however, most patients decide at the first visit to have the test, having given the test some thought before they even come to the clinic. In a minority of patients it may be best to postpone the test. For instance, in the case of a physically well homosexual man whose partner died of AIDS six months previously, and who is now depressed and abuses alcohol daily because of the fear of HIV disease, the correct initial steps are to withdraw him from alcohol, give psychotherapy and possibly antidepressants later on, and to return to the issue of HIV disease when his mental state has improved.

In spite of pretest counselling about a third of all patients who are told of their HIV positivity develop a short-lived grief reaction. Half of these will go on to a more protracted reaction lasting weeks or months, suffering all or some of the symptoms of anxiety, depression, hypochondriasis, fatigue, and lethergy. As the latter symptoms overlap with those of advanced HIV disease, careful physical and psychological assessment is mandatory.

It is now generally accepted that HIV subacute encephalopathy and its associated dementia are unlikely to develop in patients until the CD4 count is low and the viral load is high. Once the patient has AIDS, psychological symptoms should be considered to be organic (pulmonary, hepatic, and renal malfunction, cerebral infections, tumours, or dementia) until organic disease is excluded. Depression is commonly found in patients with AIDS. Loss of health and youthful looks, financial worries and dying itself are but some of the issues that may underlie the depression. Most HIV centres now have psychiatrists with a special interest in the management of these problems.

Since the advent of combination chemotherapy for HIV disease, it is the anecdotal experience of many physicians that the return of good health, and confidence in the efficacy of the therapy has resulted in a number of patients returning to high-risk sexual activity.

Marital and sexual dysfunction

Most patients with sexual dysfunction who attend STD clinics are self-referred, and probably seek the anonymity and confidentiality that the clinic affords. Many clinics offer treatment for erectile dysfunction, but limit themselves in treatment to the organic approach. However, most are sympathetic to the wide spectrum of sexual problems. A small number offer a wide service for sexual dysfunction with a multidisciplinary team on site, including GUM physicians, nurse practitioners, psychologists, and access to urological surgeons. In GUM clinics 25% of men and 10% of women admit to sexual dysfunction.

Treatment options for erectile dysfunction in GUM clinics

- Intracorporeal injections (alprostadil, papaverine)
- Intraurethral alprostadil ("MUSE")
- Oral (yohimbine, sildenafil (a very effective treatment available in 1999)
- Suction devices
- Cognitive and behaviour therapy
- Sensate focus
- Treatment of underlying conditions (depression, anxiety, phobias, marital problems)
- Sexual education

Many clinics run by physicians only also manage premature ejaculation, which may be primary (usually psychogenic) or secondary (eg associated with prostatitis or neurological conditions). It may be treated by cognitive

behaviour therapy, SSRI antidepressants, or cautious use of local anaesthetic creams. It is not the remit to discuss other sexual problems here, but only to discuss them as they relate to patients who attend for general STD screening. Decreased sexual desire can lead the partner or the patient (feeling his/her condition is primarily due to the partner) to have sex outside the relationship. Problems with arousal (erection in the man) can lead to similar results, as can retarded orgasm in either sex. Vaginismus may be primary (usually psychogenic) or secondary (eg to severe first-attack genital herpes, rape) or may be due to a recently recognised condition called vestibulitis, which causes patchy very tender hyperaemia in the vestibule (and biopsy proven acute inflammatory change) and severe burning pain exacerbated by sexual intercourse. It may cause secondary vaginismus and may be diagnosed by finding small areas of extreme tenderness in the vestibule ellicited by touching with a cotton bud—the "cotton bud test". Vaginismus of all aetiologies may present in the clinic when speculum insertion is attempted.

Marital and relationship problems can underlie having sexual intercourse outside the long-term relationship. Some patients may be unable to make such relationships and therefore only have casual sex rather than sex within a relationship. Sexual closeness is only one type of intimacy. Others include physical intimacy (eg, grooming), emotional intimacy (shared feelings), and operational intimacy (shared problems). Defects in the latter three may be a cause for overusing the sexual factor, but psychological and psychiatric factors are also important.

Underage sex, rape and sexual assault

Girls below the age of 16 and homosexual men below the age of 18 are often seen in clinics for routine screening of STDs. The legal requirement to disclose consenting underage sex must be balanced by the physician's concern for patient confidentiality. Such disclosure to the authorities of underage sexual acts will discourage the patient, and by word of mouth other such patients from attending GUM departments. This may have disasterous consequences in terms of spread of infection in the community. When in doubt about the patient's ability to understand the relevant issues or the presence of psychological problems, the hospital's legal adviser or a defence union should be consulted before proceeding.

One in four women and one in ten men admit to being raped, sexually assaulted or to being a victim of attempted sexual assault. Most assailants are known to their victims. It is vital to treat such patients with the utmost speed, sympathy, and efficiency. Some clinics have code names, for example "the Tulip clinic", so that reception staff immediately know to "fast track" the

patient. Patients should see a doctor of the sex of their choosing, which will normally be a female in the case of a woman who has been raped. However, the most senior doctor should be available to give advice at the time, and for medicolegal reasons because he/she probably has the most experience with the emotional aspects of assault. The forensic examination, gathering of specimens to exclude infection, and treatment prophylaxis are beyond the remit of this chapter. In the acute phase after these events most patients have high anxiety levels and may be fearful of dying. However, some acutely traumatised patients appear outwardly very relaxed and normal. Most of the psychological symptoms in the days and weeks following the event will be similar to those of anxiety and depression, but also include "flashbacks", intrusive thoughts, and relationship and sexual problems. Intervention and follow up by an experienced psychologist is mandatory. About a third of patients recover in months, a third take years and a further third are still symptomatic after four to six years.

METHODS OF CONTROL

Education and information

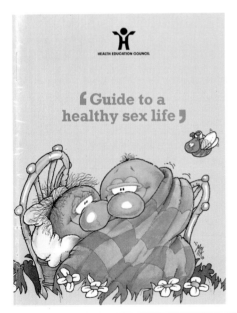

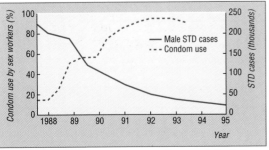

Rising condom use by sexual workers and declining STD's in Thailand 1988–95

The STDs represent one of the major health problems in the world today. The size of the problem has been referred to earlier (see first chapter). The demographic, sociological, economic, and behavioural changes seen throughout the world in the past 30 years will continue to contribute towards an even greater problem in controlling sexually acquired infections in the future. The advent of human immunodeficiency virus (HIV) infection and AIDS has highlighted the importance of good control programmes for the STDs. In general those countries with an efficient service for these diseases have found it easier to control the HIV–AIDS epidemic.

The approach to the control of STDs and emphasis placed on different components will depend on whether one is working in a resource-rich or -poor country, and the cultural mores found in these different settings.

Education of the public and health care workers is an important control measure. Society cannot continue to remain ambivalent about health education for sexually transmitted diseases. There is no evidence that widely available information about these diseases (or about contraception) encourages immoral or promiscuous behaviour.

Primary prevention should aim at educating individuals about the advantages of discriminate and safe sex and prophylaxis. It has to be accepted, however, that there is no agreement in most societies about what constitutes "normal" sexual behaviour. The skilled educator acknowledges this and constructs information that allows an individual, whatever his or her beliefs, to identify with some, if not all, of what is said. Education about sexually transmitted diseases should cover a wide range of sexual attitudes and behaviour. The best way to avoid sexually transmitted disease is to avoid sexual intercourse. This may not, however, be acceptable to those already sexually active, and they may want to know that monogamous sexual intercourse will cut down the risk. Again, this message may not be acceptable, but it should be pointed out that changing partners often increases greatly the risk of contracting diseases. Awareness of the presenting symptoms of the common diseases is important, but it is also important to point out that disease can be asymptomatic and that regular check ups (every three months) are a wise precaution for those changing their partners often. The use of a barrier contraceptive will reduce the risk of certain diseases and is a wise prophylactic measure when changing sexual partners. The sheath may, however, give a false sense of security.

The importance of the condom has been emphasised in the past few years particularly in relation to HIV infection. Health education can work, as witnessed by a decline in syphilis and gonorrhoea among homosexual men who originally modified their sexual behaviour in the light of the HIV epidemic.

The advent of AIDS has had a major influence on increasing the awareness of the need for health education and the public acceptance of explicit messages and images. Programmes to market and

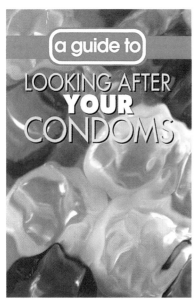

Reproduced with permission from Durex

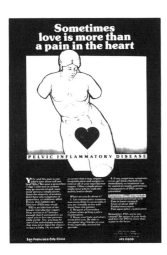

encourage the use of condoms (social marketing) have been at the heart of many control programmes in countries such as Thailand, Zimbabwe, Uganda, etc, and are particularly useful because they reduce acquisition and transmission of both traditional STDs and HIV infection. In Africa and Thailand there has been encouraging evidence that increased condom use has been accepted by high-risk groups such as commercial sex workers and their clients, and that this has altered levels of infection.

In resource-poor countries, social, cultural and economic issues also need to be addressed. Often women are so poor and disempowered that they have sex on a commercial basis against their will and are unable to effectively negotiate the use of condoms by clients. Women need to be taught skills that help them negotiate safer sex with clients and regular partners. This is particularly difficult with the latter, because husbands and regular partners can see such negotiation as a reflection of themselves, at the same time as suggesting that the woman has herself had multiple partners. Thus, substantial shifts in cultural attitudes and the role of women will be necessary for the effective control of both STDs and HIV infection.

Secondary prevention aims at encouraging people to seek care without delay once the symptoms of a disease are recognised, stop sexual intercourse until medical advice has been sought, and adhere to the advice given.

Since STD is such a major health problem, more resources need to be devoted towards health education and making the public aware of clinics. Facilities should be advertised in places frequented more readily and openly by the public and not furtively in public toilets.

Early diagnosis and treatment are cheap; late sequelae of untreated disease are expensive. For example, if a good control programme exists most cases of pelvic inflammatory disease are preventable; if not prevented, however, the psychological, social, and monetary costs are large. Such costs increase further with developments in medical technology; thus, fallopian tube microsurgery and in vitro fertilisation and implantation of human embryos can now be performed at great expense in those sterilised by pelvic inflammatory disease. Prevention is better than cure, which is better than late intervention.

There are several complementary ways in which STDs can be controlled. In the UK the most important way is through health promotion and the provision of adequate diagnostic and treatment facilities in departments of genitourinary medicine. The aims of this service are to offer prompt diagnosis and treatment, minimise the incidence of complications, trace and treat the infected partners of patients, and educate patients, the public, and healthcare workers.

Reducing the risk of contracting a sexually transmitted disease

(1) Abstain

(2) Avoid multiple partners, prostitutes, and other people with multiple sex partners

(3) Avoid sexual contact with people who have symptoms or lesions (eg urethral discharge, warts, ulcers)

(4) Avoid genital contact with oral "cold sores"

(5) Use condoms or diaphragm

(6) Have regular check ups if at high risk of sexually transmitted disease

---

Aims of genitourinary medicine

- Prompt diagnosis and treatment
- Minimise incidence of complications and disability
- Trace and treat sexual contacts
- Education

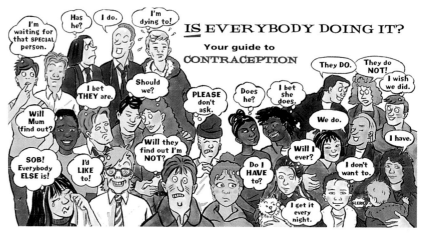

Reproduced with permission from the Family Planning Association.

Clinics

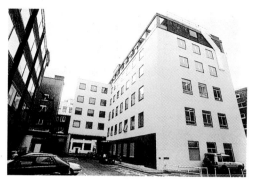

Genitourinary clinics should be accessible and alleviate stigma.

There are 240 departments of genitourinary medicine/sexually transmitted diseases/sexual health in the UK. Most clinics are situated within a general hospital, in the outpatient department or in their own purpose built premises. Unfortunately, some are still found in dingy basements or down dark alleyways. Facilities should alleviate, not create, stigma and be readily accessible for self referral. Some departments are called after physicians, apostles, or battles and others are termed "Special department" or given a number or letter. These differences make it difficult for patients to find their bearings and only add to their alienation, presenting a further hurdle to consultation. The official title for the specialty and its clinics is genitourinary medicine. Other terms such as STDs and sexual health are also used.

People looking after patients with STDs should use language that is easily understood by the patient, including slang when appropriate. Healthcare staff may well have different moral and sexual attitudes from their patients. They have to accept and come to terms with this and their own sexuality before being able to cope with patients. It is bad manners for staff to force their own attitudes on a patient and it is also bad medicine, since the patient will not come back.

Contact tracing

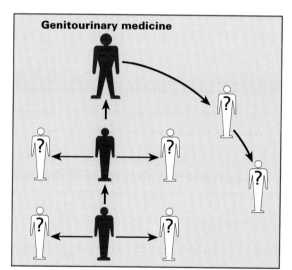

Tracing sexual contacts is an essential part of a control programme. Interviewing patients about their contacts requires tact, sensitivity, and special communication skills. For any one patient (index case) presenting to a clinic there are at least two other people affected—the person who infected the patient and the person who infected that contact. It is usually more complicated than this, so that by the time the index patient has sought medical care he or she may have had intercourse with a further individual. It is essential, therefore, to get in touch as soon as possible with sexual contacts and advise them to attend a clinic. The aim is to control the disease within the community as well as to protect the health of individuals who are symptomless and unaware of their disease. For women with gonococcal and chlamydial infections the prevention of costly disability is of paramount importance.

Some patients feel that being asked about contacts is unnecessary or an infringement of their privacy. The reasons for tracing contacts must be explained to the patient and their active cooperation sought. Often this is a useful health education exercise.

How a patient is managed

Any doctor may refer a patient to a department of genitourinary medicine for diagnosis or treatment or to ensure contact tracing. The earlier chapters have given guidelines on how to recognise and diagnose disease and which patients to refer. Physicians working in departments of genitourinary medicine are always happy to see any patient in whom an STD is suspected or needs to be excluded.

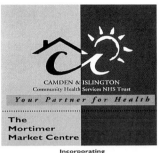

Patients may be extremely anxious about their condition, talking about sexual matters, and what investigations will be performed. Some of these fears can be modified if the person referring the patient can explain how a clinic works.

Finding a clinic—Most patients refer themselves to clinics and often know of a clinic through friends or sexual contacts, or they may be referred by a general practitioner or family planning clinic. Otherwise, information about STD clinics can be obtained in most large cities from recorded messages and telephone directories. In recent years magazines have printed articles about the STDs and given star ratings to some clinics and crossed wooden spoons to others. Information of this sort helps patients to find out where the clinics are and the quality of service they may expect.

Some clinics have an appointments system, and a new patient gets an appointment, usually within 24–48 hours, by ringing or visiting the clinic. Other clinics have no appointments and simply invite patients to walk in and be seen. Some run a combined system.

What happens in a clinic

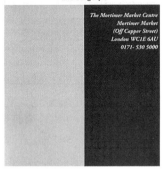

Example of a patient registration form

New patients have to register in the clinic. Most clinics have a record system separate from that of the main hospital to ensure confidentiality, and patients do not have to give any personal or demographic details, though few refuse. Then, if laboratory tests are positive and a patient fails to keep an appointment he or she can be told of the results and of the importance of attending. If a patient specifically requests no correspondence, this is respected.

The consultation—Details of the presenting symptoms and their duration are taken and information elicited to exclude possible complications—for example, abdominal pain, arthralgia. Patients will be asked about the occurrence and timing of symptoms in relation to sexual exposure and menstruation, the type of contraception used, the number of recent sexual contacts and whether any of these have symptoms and have received treatment. The sexual orientation of the patient is important. Homosexual patients do not always volunteer this information, particularly if they are under 18 and think that the doctor will report them to the police. If the patient is homosexual he will be asked about the sites put at risk of infection. Finally, a history of previous STD and sensitivity to antibiotics will be obtained from all patients and, in women, details of any menstrual changes, pregnancies, and recent gynaecological procedures and cervical cytology.

MORTIMER MARKET CENTRE
Mortimer Market
London, WC1E 6AU

Tel: 0171-530 5050

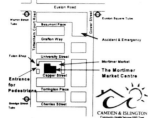

Open:	Mon	9.00a.m. - 6.00p.m.
	Tues	9.00a.m. - 11.00a.m.
		3.45p.m. - 7.00p.m.
	Wed	9.00a.m. - 6.00p.m.
	Thurs	9.00a.m. - 6.00p.m.
	fri	9.00a.m. - 2.45p.m.

On receipt of this slip we strongly advise you to make an appointment as soon as possible by ringing **0171-530 5050**, Monday - Friday.

If you would like to speak to a health professional, in confidence, about this slip please ring **0171-530 5111**.

This is a free and confidential service.

> **PLEASE BRING THIS SLIP WITH YOU WHEN YOU ATTEND AND GIVE TO THE DOCTOR**

Example of a contact tracing slip

The examination—A local genital examination is carried out and selectively or routinely augmented by a general physical examination. *Women* are usually examined in the lithotomy position and the external genitalia examined for evidence of disease. Specimens for microscopy and culture are taken from the posterior fornix, vaginal wall, endocervix, and urethra (see chapter on vaginal discharge). Cervical cytology may also be performed. In selected patients proctoscopy is performed and specimens taken (if the patient is a contact of someone with gonorrhoea or volunteers anal or rectal symptoms). This is followed by a bimanual examination. Serological tests for syphilis are performed in all patients since this can be a concurrent asymptomatic infection. Additional tests—haemoglobin, midstream urine, throat swab—are performed if indicated. Finally, urine is tested for protein and sugar. Microscopy can be performed immediately in the clinic and in most cases a diagnosis obtained. If this is not always possible—for example in women—the need to culture specimens is explained and patients are asked to return in three to seven days. In *men* general physical and local genital examinations are performed and samples obtained. Anal examination and proctoscopy and sampling are carried out when indicated. In homosexuals samples are taken from the sites related to the symptoms or, if asymptomatic, from the sites at risk. As in women, serological tests for syphilis, urine tests, and any necessary additional tests are performed. Testing for antibodies to HIV is performed only after counselling and consent.

Treatment—If a STD is diagnosed microscopically within the clinic the patient will be given treatment at once. All treatment is free of prescription charges.

Contact tracing will be undertaken by a contact tracer (social health adviser) or patient who can visit or telephone contacts. Contact slips are still used, but with the wider availability of telephones they are no longer so popular. A contact slip will be given to the contact(s) by the patient or health adviser. This can be taken to any clinic in the UK. The slip includes the original patient's note number and a code for the diagnosis. This diagnosis is vital information for the doctor seeing the contact and will help him decide on the appropriate tests. If the contact is seen at a different clinic from the index case the slip will be returned to the original clinic so that accurate contact tracing records can be kept.

Confidentiality

The confidentiality of information imparted by patients to doctors or contact tracers is paramount in the practice of genitourinary medicine. Failure to keep confidences will dissuade patients from seeking attention or volunteering information about their sexual orientation and contacts. It is essential that patients should realise that their diagnosis or, indeed, any other information is never given to their sexual partners when they consult or to any one else outside the clinic. Family practitioners are informed of the diagnosis and treatment if the patient has been referred by them in the first instance. Any inquiries, for example from solicitors or doctors performing life assurance examinations, are not answered unless the patient gives written permission. A record keeping system separate from the rest of the hospital secures the confidential nature of information. The police are never given information, even if the patient is a minor, unless the patient requests it.

The developing world

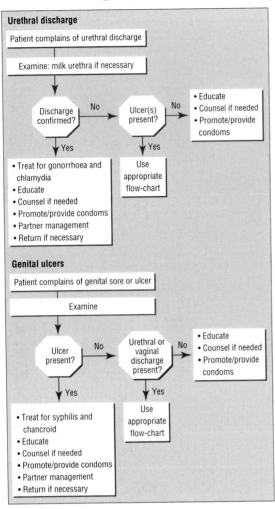

Urethral discharge

Patient complains of urethral discharge

↓

Examine: milk urethra if necessary

↓

Discharge confirmed? → No → Ulcer(s) present? → No → • Educate • Counsel if needed • Promote/provide condoms

↓ Yes

• Treat for gonorrhoea and chlamydia
• Educate
• Counsel if needed
• Promote/provide condoms
• Partner management
• Return if necessary

Ulcer(s) present? ↓ Yes → Use appropriate flow-chart

Genital ulcers

Patient complains of genital sore or ulcer

↓

Examine

↓

Ulcer present? → No → Urethral or vaginal discharge present? → No → • Educate • Counsel if needed • Promote/provide condoms

↓ Yes

• Treat for syphilis and chancroid
• Educate
• Counsel if needed
• Promote/provide condoms
• Partner management
• Return if necessary

Urethral or vaginal discharge present? ↓ Yes → Use appropriate flow-chart

Algorithms for urethral discharge and genital ulceration

Models of case management so far described for use in resource-rich countries are usually inappropriate for implementation in developing countries in which such care is provided through a whole array of services and individuals, usually not medically qualified, complemented by pharmacists, traditional healers, quacks, and street vendors.

A specialist-based approach, often in urban centres with laboratory support, is not appropriate or cost effective. The World Health Organisation has placed increasing emphasis on integrated systems, especially at the rural primary healthcare level, using a syndromic approach for patient management. The syndromic approach uses algorithms based upon commonly presenting signs and symptoms, for example genital ulcer, urethral and vaginal discharge, where laboratory support may or may not be present. The algorithm for genital ulcers works on the basic premise that the two commonest causes of such a sign/symptom are syphilis and chancroid, and with no laboratory support and the difficulty in establishing an accurate clinical diagnosis, it is appropriate to give therapy for both conditions. Likewise, the algorithm for urethral discharge assumes that the aetiology could be gonococcal and/or chlamydial, and that therapy appropriate for both should be utilised. A recent study from Tanzania has demonstrated the importance and effect of an integrated STD programme in rural communities on HIV incidence. This randomised controlled trial showed that improved STD care integrated at primary care level resulted in a reduction of HIV incidence of 42% over the two-year period of the study. The study confirms the effects of STDs on HIV acquisition and transmission and that the integrated non-specialist and syndromic approach can be very effective.

INDEX

Index